Healing Scripts
Using Hypnosis to Treat Trauma and Stress

Marlene E. Hunter MD

Crown House Publishing Limited
www.crownhouse.co.uk
www.chpus.com

First published by

Crown House Publishing Ltd
Crown Buildings, Bancyfelin, Carmarthen, Wales, SA33 5ND, UK
www.crownhouse.co.uk

and

Crown House Publishing Company LLC
6 Trowbridge Drive, Suite 5, Bethel, CT 06801-2858, USA
www.CHPUS.com

British Library Cataloguing-in-Publication Data
A catalogue entry for this book is available
from the British Library.

ISBN 978-184590072-4

LCCN 2007925538

Printed and bound by
Cromwell Press, Trowbridge, Wiltshire

Dedication

As always, for Redner, with love.

Contents

Introduction vii

Section I: Pain..1
  Hypnosis and the relief of pain...1
    Pain and dissociation 1
  Mind–body communication 5
    Somatoform dissociation...9
  Pain as a dissociative experience 13
    Emotional pain..13
    Physical pain..15
    Physiological pain 17
    Organic pain...19
    Flashback pain 21
    Chronic pain..24
    Chronic pain syndrome..26

Section II: Stress Disorders...31
  Post-Traumatic Stress Disorder 31
    Denial 31
    Hypervigilance 36
    Hyperarousal 41
    Lack of trust 45
    Flashbacks 51
    Sleep flashbacks..55
    Other sleep disorders...59
  Acute Traumatic Stress Disorder 77
    Self-worth 84
    Physiological response to trauma..86
  Critical Incident Stress Disorder 90
  Obsessive-Compulsive Disorder 93
  Anxiety disorders..97
    Reactive anxiety..97
    Conditioned anxiety 99
    Free-floating anxiety 102
  Panic attacks...105
  Phobias...107
  Depression...110
  Grief and bereavement..112
    Children 116
    Palliative care..117

Section III: Dissociative Disorders..**119**

   Safety—inside and out 119

      Helping the child part to tell...122

      Ego strengthening 131

      Getting along together—inside..138

   Blending...140

      Getting along together—outside...143

      More about blending 145

   Integration or resolution?..148

      Preparing for resolution 148

      More about preparation for resolution 150

      Preparing for integration 156

Section IV: Children..**159**

   For the teenager...165

References...171

Index 173

Introduction

The idea of writing a book about the use of hypnosis when working with clients who have suffered severe trauma has been niggling away in the back of my mind for many years. After the publication of *Understanding Dissociative Disorders: A Guide for Family Physicians and Health Care Professionals*, the need for such a book became much clearer. In particular, the need for such a book specifically for those who have had training and experience both in clinical hypnosis and in working with what are now called "trauma-spectrum disorders" became almost a mission.

To my knowledge, there is no other book on the use of clinical hypnosis that is dedicated to this specialty—that of helping men and women (and, of course, children) who have suffered and are still suffering from the effects of child abuse, or those who have experienced dreadful trauma through wars and other disasters, and who still live with it in their day-to-day lives.

We need to recognize several aspects of this work:

- It is specialized, and demands specialized training and experience
- Those who suffer from these traumata are particularly vulnerable to misinterpretations and/or subliminal messages from past events
- The healing of trauma always takes time, and the length of time is different for each person that we, as psychotherapists, encounter in our practices
- Those who have suffered trauma are very vulnerable

It is because of the vulnerability of this client group that it is essential that the therapists are well-trained in all aspects of their approach: this includes recognizing and becoming proficient in the various therapeutic approaches that are helpful, and by-passing those approaches which could cause more harm than good or in which they do not have sufficient experience.

I had already been doing clinical hypnosis for several years before I met my first Multiple Personality Disorder client. Indeed, my training in clinical hypnosis was the reason that my colleague, a family physician who was moving out of town, asked me if I would take this woman into my family practice. The client, whom I will call "Jayere" because that is what I have called her in previous publications, was having terrible headaches, and my colleague thought that continuing hypnosis—which she (the colleague) had been doing—might be helpful.

You may have read about Jayere in other publications or heard about her at conferences, because I have spoken about her many times. She, and two other dissociative clients whom I subsequently realized that I had in my family practice, taught me all of the basics about working with the long-term effects of childhood trauma. Of particular importance for this book, however, is the work with hypnosis in the context of traumatized clients—especially, although not only, those who were so miserably treated when they were young.

It is always important to use hypnosis carefully within the professional milieu. (Of course, it is always important to use it carefully, period, but not all entertainment hypnotists spend time recognizing that—which has led to many a lawsuit.)

Employing hypnosis as a therapeutic tool with clients who have endured trauma, however, takes the need for careful appraisal one big step further. Many, if not all, people who have a dissociative disorder or Post-Traumatic Stress Disorder or for that matter any significant psychosomatic problem, are particularly vulnerable to the possibility of being catapulted back into the traumatic situation while in an altered state of consciousness. This can lead to difficulties along many lines—exacerbating the traumatic response, for example, or creating an unsought and certainly unwanted new dilemma regarding veracity. In this regard, I had exceptional good luck, because these three clients from my own family practice, who knew me, undertook my education! And in many ways, they protected me from making huge mistakes.

It is because of the potential problems that I have written this book. Its various sections attend to pain in many of its various intrusions; to post-traumatic stress disorders, its seven main symptoms, and the precursors of these: critical incidents and acute traumatic stress disorders; dissociative disorders including dissociative identity disorder (which used to be called Multiple Personality Disorder); the concept of ego states (parts of the personality structure that have specific tasks in the system); other dissociative disorders not so well defined—Dissociative Disorder Not Otherwise Specified, as the DSM (Diagnostic and Statistical Manual) describes it; grief, especially the kind of deep grieving that does not abate with time but becomes a major psychological difficulty; and a special section on children who have been, or are still being, abused.

You will realize early on that many scripts are very basic indeed, or are simply ways to introduce a hypnotic intervention rather than a fulfilling word-by-word description. Other scripts are more complete, and some have alternative language suggestions. But the basic point is: *never* attempt to use hypnosis with trauma-spectrum disorders until you are very well schooled in the use of clinical hypnosis. That, at least, I did have when Jayere came so unexpectedly onto my horizon. And the same caution is required for those who offer psychotherapy for such clients. Professional education is a must.

Luckily, I became a member of the International Society for the Study of Multiple Personality and Dissociation at its very first meeting in Chicago in 1984, several years after my "training" by Jayere and the other two clients in my practice had begun. Subsequently that organization became ISSD (International Society for the Study of Dissociation) and now ISSTD (add Trauma to the name). Although I had learned a great deal from my clients, I needed professional help and found it in those organizations. Other countries have similar organizations—seek them out. And also seek out professional organizations for education in clinical hypnosis, if you have not done that already.

I sold my family practice in 1989 because the work with trauma disorders had overtaken my work as a family physician. Rather than attempt to do three things, and maybe do them badly, it was more important to focus on the two that were so in need of trained professionals. I miss family medicine, but am not sorry that I decided to shift my focus. The subsequent years have brought their own rewards

If the client has never done hypnosis before, then it is important for them to have some introductory sessions on basic relaxation techniques before starting on specific situations such as those described in this book.

I hope that you find this book useful. Hypnosis is a wonderful tool, but sometimes we forget that it *is* a tool, not magic.

Section I

Pain

Hypnosis and the relief of pain

For many decades, hypnosis as a means to relieve pain has been a very useful tool. Pain, itself, is a common experience in all walks of life and in all ages and populations. Pain can be a warning signal that something is wrong—injury, infection or a severe allergic response during which the person cannot easily take a breath. In all of these situations, hypnosis, when carefully done by a therapist who is well-trained in the various hypnotic techniques, can bring comfort.

Pain that is part of (or the result of) various kinds of trauma, however, has an added component—one that is important for us to recognize. That component is the emotional response to the *situation* in which the pain is experienced, or from which it is derived. The use of hypnosis as one—but only one—of the techniques that can be useful in psychotherapy is exemplified in the following scripts. Perhaps the client (or the therapist) is feeling stuck for some reason; perhaps the emotional aspect has become too intrusive or needs to be recognized. A session, or several sessions, of hypnosis may open the gate again, offering new insights or alternative ways of managing the situation.

Pain and dissociation

Pain is a dissociative experience. It can be dissociative in the sense that we put distance between ourselves and how we are experiencing the sensation itself, which is what we might do in the dentist's chair. It could also mean that we distance ourselves from what is going on around us and focus instead on the pain. The former is useful insofar as it alleviates the physical discomfort; the second, however, could precipitate far more distress than one would ordinarily expect in any given situation.

When the latter occurs, careful hypnosis can be very helpful. We need to remember the role of hypnosis in relieving pain. It is not that hypnosis causes pain to disappear—often it doesn't do that at all. What it *does* do is to help put some distance between the self and the pain, so that the pain per se doesn't matter so much. The client is no longer so bothered by the pain and can therefore get on with whatever is happening in their life.

There are also situations during which the dissociation from pain is crucial—for example, there is a fire and the most important thing is to get the children out of the house. The sensation of pain is disregarded because the children take 100% precedence. However, later on, when the children are (hopefully) safe, then the sensation of pain can be overwhelming, even to the point where others cannot understand *why* it should be so overwhelming. It is so because the emotional aspect of the situation ("my children are in danger") is then superimposed on the physical pain, even though the danger is no longer there. It is as if the subconscious is saying, "but what if—but what if—", over and over again.

It is important to find out as much as possible regarding the origin of the pain. We need to remember that the client's perception of the origin of the pain may not be the true origin of the pain. Does the dissociation mask an important part of the pain which would be crucial to an appropriate diagnosis? These are aspects that may need to be discussed with the family doctor or specialist, with the client's permission.

Does the client's lifestyle exacerbate mental or emotional pain? Are they in financial crisis? In trouble with the law? Alone, with no support from, for example, an estranged family? Are they ignoring another—possibly important—physical problem?

How we, as physicians and/or therapists, approach these possible problems may have a profound impact on the future health—emotional *and* physical—of the client.

Taking all of this into consideration, make the initial hypnotic intervention very generic, rather than explicit. The following two scripts describe this.

First script

Jane, we have talked about the misery of the pain you experience when (*carefully refer to the situation(s) that Jane has described in as few words as possible*) Would you like to explore a possible helpful solution? (*Yes*)

Setting the scene

Offering a possible escape

Alright, then just settle into your hypnosis, as you know how to do, knowing that you are here, safe in my office. Let me know when you reach the level of hypnosis that you think would be useful today. (*Signals*)

"Here, safe in my office ..." is very important

Good. Now, begin to create a wonderful, safe barrier or shield of some kind, around you. It could be a cloud, or a colour, or warm, or music, or a magic fence—whatever you just instinctively know is the right one for you. Let me know when you have done that. (*Signals*)

This is the important suggestion, offering possible ways to do this

That's right. And now that you know that you are safe behind that wonderful barrier of your own choice, *now* you can allow yourself to recognize that pain, while knowing all the time that you have that strong, safe barrier between you and the experience of that past discomfort. Let me know when you have allowed that to happen, *under your own control*. (*Signals*)

She now has created her own safety shield, not somebody else's shield

Shifting to the word "discomfort" will alter the perception

Excellent. You can stay there, in that same experience, for a few more moments—as long as you like in hypnosis time but just a very short time by clock time. That's right. Good.

Now, in your own way, do what you need to do to make the uncomfortable situation dissolve, and then let me know when have done that. You will still be safely behind your protective barrier or shield. (*Signals*)

She can do it herself

Still protected—very important

Excellent. And you can appreciate your own strength, in the way you managed that situation. And now you know that you can do that.

"... your own strength ..." gives her the sense of self-sufficiency

When I make the suggestion, you can bring yourself out of hypnosis in your own way.

Second script

(Note: Whilst the first script, above, has to do with safety, this one offers more variations, for example, a metaphor or simile that is appropriate for the client. The one below is offered as an example, with the suggestion that the client consider further possibilities that are specific for him.)

Jim, it seems as if you need a more specific type of suggestion, one that is personal for you, to get you started. Is that right? (*Nods*)	**Offering another possibility**
That makes sense for you, so find out if this suggestion could help. You can go into hypnosis, or just close your eyes and take the suggestion into your mind, to ponder on it, when and how you choose.	**Many people will go into a light trance anyhow, when offered this opportunity**
Some people find that they can link the pain with similes that relate to their own past experiences. For example, you might say to yourself, "This pain is like a vise, gripping me just like the vise in my home workshop grips the (*wood, metal, etc.*) that I am working with. It is very, very strong, and feels like it will never let me go.	**Offering a specific example**
But you are also aware that, when you are ready to do so, you can release the pressure in the vise so that you can extract the (*wood, metal,* etc.) and begin to work with the object, maybe to fine-tune it, or to give it a finishing polish.	**Making the connection between the simile and the situation**
You can do the same sort of thing— releasing the pressure—when the intense discomfort becomes too much. Just work with the *internal pressure* in the same way that you would work with the object in the vise.	**Adapting the simile to the real situation**
As I said at the beginning, it is important that the simile you use has meaning for you personally, so experiment, and next week we can work a little further in this direction.	**Very important!**

Mind–body communication

Of all the things we know (but maybe used not to know), one stands out clearly: we are never disconnected at the neck.

Pain has many components; two of the most obvious are the physiological component and the emotional component. These are inextricably joined. At times the physiological response is foremost, at other times the emotions take precedence in the awareness and response of the person.

Many years ago, at a meeting in Vancouver, Dr. Barry Wyke, a neurophysiologist from the UK, offered this opinion: "Pain is an emotion". It created quite a stir in the room as it was immediately interpreted as meaning "… and therefore not real". The immediate implication, to many in the room, was that "emotion" was equated with the pain being unimportant or even malingering. He did *not* mean that; what he meant was that our minds, as well as our bodies, were responding to the awareness of pain.

In fact, pain can indeed be equated with emotion, if one recognizes the close relationship between mind and body. We respond to pain, and we respond emotionally, perceptually and with immediate mind–body interaction.

What happens in our minds—emotions, thought processes, perceptions, the five senses—is always reflected in our bodies. In the same way, what happens in our bodies is always reflected and recorded in our minds.

When the happenings in either mind or body are significantly important, they are routed or re-routed into one of the impressive mental libraries of experience and learning. And from there they can be elicited and interpreted, perhaps in new ways or as reflections of the past.

Some of the most important of all those happenings have to do with pain—be it emotional, psychological or physical. It may be a moot point as to whether the mind or the body was the first to recognize that pain; the results are the same—the mind–body communication between the conscious (cognitive, left brain), the subconscious (perceptual, right brain) and the body. Although the "left brain, right brain" distinction is too simplistic it does offer a perspective that people find useful.

All injury is traumatic to some degree. That degree depends on the depth of the intrusion and interference that the injury causes, or of the previous experience it may subsequently bring back into focus.

Often we are unaware, cognitively, what that previous injury may have been; at other times, we know, but may we be hard put to do anything about it.

Because of all these layers of mind–body communication, and because of the possible emotional scars that may be in place, we need to be particularly careful when using hypnosis to ameliorate the distress. It is a great tool but must be understood and activated in very careful ways. Generally, the less we say, and the more we allow the client to find their own path, the better. We are, however, there to guide, and that guidance is crucial.

Influencing the mind–body connection

(Tom has been suffering from chronic post-viral fatigue syndrome which started with an upper respiratory infection two years before.)

Today we are going to discuss, in more detail, some of the many ways in which mind and body work together. It is a truly miraculous partnership, and one that we can utilize even more fully, in hypnosis.	**Recognizing the importance and offering better opportunities for success**
Get very comfortably settled, then, in your own way, taking yourself a little further into hypnosis to that level which you instinctively know is just right for you at this time. You know that you *can always change* your level of hypnosis—deeper or lighter—*whenever that change would be useful* for you.	*"You can always change … whenever that change would be useful"*; **multilevel meaning— alter vocal tone accordingly**
Turn your attention to your own body, now, and to what has been happening to it during these past two years. It has been a very distressing and discouraging time; now you feel within yourself that you are beginning to get well again. We want to foster that process by encouraging your mind and body to work together in the most positive way.	**Stating the fact** **Respect intuition** **How to proceed**

We have talked about the fact that chronic stress depresses the immune defenses of the body, and these past two years certainly have been stressful for you. So we will begin by focusing on the body's immune system.

Validating the long illness

Go even further within yourself now, to the very center of yourself, and ask your subconscious mind and your body to communicate, *each giving the other the information it needs* for your immune system defenses to become strong and vital again. Your subconscious mind and your body *together* can communicate, collaborate, cooperate and do *whatever needs to be done* to achieve that return to strong healthy function.

The communication is always "bidirectional" (Rossi, 1986)

Alliterative emphasis

That's right. *Feel* that communication occurring, at your deepest intuitive level. Good. Very, very good. As your defenses become stronger and stronger, you know that you are protected from further infection, and so you can direct more energy to healing and restoring within your body.

Kinaesthetic awareness

Good things are happening, which lead to more good things

Strength begins to return to your muscles, your appetite improves and you sleep better.

Ask your subconscious mind and your body to communicate on all these aspects, also, during your own hypnosis time every day, and in the same way, to do *whatever needs to be done* to achieve this return to health. Add your own healing imagery to this practical and effective convalescent program.

The subconscious and the body together know what needs to be done; you can further the process with healing imagery

And with healing comes a lifting of those feelings of depression. You *know* that you are getting better, and it is wonderfully reassuring to know that.

The process continues

Everything we say, or think; everything
we *feel*, every emotion; how we behave,
and why we behave that way—all of these
are directly translated into some response
within the body. This is vital information
for us when we are considering mind–
body communication.

Mind–body communication

Therefore let yourself become *even more*
aware of your thoughts and words and
actions; and if you discover, for instance,
that you are speaking in a negative way ("I
don't feel well"), then you can change that
immediately to a positive statement ("I'll
feel better tomorrow"). This reinforces, for
your subconscious mind, the message that
positive is what you intend.

**Suggestion for deepening now as
well as greater awareness later**

How to utilize

Best of all is the knowledge that your
mind and body are working together,
a true partnership; and that you can
enhance that partnership through your
own resources and your own hypnosis
every day.*

You are important!

Another useful suggestion is the following concept:

> You can think of the communication between your mind and your body as
> being part of a triangle: top of the triangle can be thought of as the brain,
> the conscious mind; then, on the left-hand side of the base we have the
> subconscious, and on the right-hand side, the body.

> Communication occurs along *all* sides of this triangle between conscious
> and subconscious, between conscious and the body, and between the
> subconscious and the body. All are important, but *the most important is the
> communication across the base*, the *subconscious–body* connection.

> This is the connection that is strengthened in your hypnosis, and why it is
> important to do your hypnosis every day.

> And remember, the communication goes both ways. There are no one-way
> streets in this land—just wonderful sharing of information, communication,
> back and forth, along all sides of the triangle. Conscious, thinking mind;
> subconscious, emotional mind; sensate, experiencing body.*

> *You.*

---

*These scripts have been reproduced from *Creative Scripts for Hypnotherapy*, by Marlene E.
Hunter, Brunner-Routledge. (1994), with permission.

To give a reinforcing post-hypnotic suggestion that will enhance these mind–body communication concepts, you might say:

> And you can ask your mind and your body to continue this communication, to collaborate and cooperate towards achieving your healing and recovery.

> And you can reinforce this for yourself many times throughout the day by just repeating this little mnemonic: "M-B-C-C-C". That's right, you can make it into a little jingle: "M-B-C-C-C". Mind–Body Communication, Collaboration, Cooperation. Say it to yourself many times a day, whenever you think of it, whatever you might be doing at the time.

> M-B-C-C-C. Many times, every day.*

Somatoform dissociation

There are many connections between pain and trauma, but perhaps the most important for this book is "somatoform dissociation". In such a disorder, the dissociativity—otherwise expressed as individual ego states—is instead expressed through somatic symptoms. "Ego states" simply refers to the part of the personality structure that takes care of certain situations. We all have ego states: I'm slightly different in the office than I am at home, different as a wife than as a mother, even slightly different with friends than with colleagues. These are some of my ego states. Luckily, they all know each other. In someone who has suffered severe child abuse—emotional, physical, sexual or some combination of these—the child develops ego states to cope with the traumatic situations. After a while, these ego states assume an independent quality. I will be speaking much more specifically about ego states in the Section 3 on Dissociative Disorders.

The phrase "somatoform dissociation" was coined by Dr Ellert Nijenhuis, of the Netherlands. His work opened up and recognized a huge omission in our knowledge of dissociative disorders—one that had never been thoroughly explored before. In so doing, it clarified many murky areas in the understanding of how past traumas, including emotional traumas, can be expressed through physical symptoms, even when the physicians would declare that "there is nothing wrong".

The first thing to recognize is that somatoform dissociation has absolutely nothing whatsoever to do with malingering. It is simply a way for the body to express that *emotion* which is such an important component of

---

*These scripts have been reproduced from *Creative Scripts for Hypnotherapy*, by Marlene E. Hunter, Brunner-Routledge. (1994), with permission.

pain. It turns out that there is a significant number of trauma survivors who are not dissociative, in the usual sense of the word, but who transfer that dissociation into an incongruity between mind and body—what the mind cognitively recognizes and what the body perceives. Put another way, the ego states assume mantles of pain as their individual identities.

These ego states and the pain which they carry are not necessarily age-related to the pain that they express. A young ego state may have pain which would ordinarily be associated with middle-aged, or even older, ego states. This becomes more relevant when working with a dissociative disorder in which the various identities are specifically described. In Dr Nijenhuis's book, *Somatoform Dissociation*, he and his colleagues describe and ascribe dissociative characteristics to physical symptoms. It is an understanding that those of us who work with dissociativity need to recognize.

In such situations, we work with the ego state experiencing the pain, whether or not it makes cognitive sense.

First script

(Jackie has been very distressed because her physician doesn't seem to understand her problems, and implies that she is over-reacting to her symptoms. No apparent cause has been found to explain her situation. Her past history is one of childhood abuse and neglect—especially neglect, as her mother implied that she was always "making it up" when she had some pain or physical symptom.)

Jackie, let's explore a different possibility. You can think of your physical discomfort as another part of your personality. You have said that it often seems as if the (symptom) has taken on a life of its own. We can now pretend that that is what has happened. Do you feel comfortable with exploring that metaphor? (*Yes*)	**Setting the guidelines** **Is it very important for her to agree to the idea**
Good. Then let yourself go into hypnosis in your own way, just to whatever level feels comfortable for you at this time. As we are exploring, you may choose to be at a lighter level, or a deeper level, whichever seems just right for this exploration.	**Whatever level she chooses, will be the right one for her at this time**

That's right. You can communicate with that wise subconscious mind in your own way. It may be a conversation, or as if you were reading a book or watching a movie, or with a group of people, observing their behaviour or their manner of moving around. You'll know what is the best situation for you.

Offering possible scenarios

Then, when you have found the right milieu, you can begin to have a conversation with that part of you which represents your pain (*or other symptom*), because it may be that your body wants to tell you something. So listen carefully, recognizing all the little hints that present an important picture for you to study— just as if you were looking at that movie, or reading that book, or being with that group of people.

This is the crux of the matter

She can explore it in her own way

And as the message begins to clarify, so your response will adapt to what the thought or message is really communicating.

Hypno-speak: she can interpret it in her own way

It may or may not take several sessions, over a period of time, to really understand that new message; but when you do, then you can begin to shift your response so that it reflects your new understanding.

More hypno-speak

And we may decide to have more sessions like this one, as you clarify more and more of your new recognitions.

This is reassurance that you won't abandon her halfway through this strange situation

Second script

For some clients, the above approach may be too difficult for them to grasp, especially if the whole concept of somatoform dissociation is new and/or unclear to them. In such a case, approach it from a more basic perspective.

Betty, we've been talking now for several weeks about the way our minds and our bodies sometimes seem to take on each other's roles. Let's explore that a little bit further.

A soft way to start the process of accepting the somatoform concept

You have had whole-body pain for a long time now and nobody seems to be able to find the cause, or to help you understand it.

This is the basic fact

You know how we sometimes say that a physical symptom or a habit or a sensation "seems to take on a life of its own". Let's pretend, for the sake of argument, that your pain comes into such a category. It should be fairly easy for you to do that, because I know that you sometimes speak of the pain as "he"—in other words, the pain seems to be a person. Do you feel comfortable with exploring that a little further? (*Yes*)

A familiar idea—and reassuring her that she is not crazy

Becoming more specific

Good. Then allow yourself to construct an image of what "he" looks like. You may have already done that, without even realizing it.

This comment can be both reassuring and validating

When you have found that image, then begin to hold a conversation with him. It may be a one-way conversation in the beginning, but will probably become a two-way discussion in time.

Some patience might be needed before this becomes comfortable

As time goes on, you could ask him what his real purpose is, or why he came to begin with, or—even more important—what needs to happen before he can move on.

The questions everybody in this situation struggle with

And as you get to know and understand each other better, you may find that the pain begins to soften a little bit. And you and he can talk about that, too.

Setting the scene for a positive change—but not until the real reason for the pain is recognized

As we are talking about somatoform dissociation, the real cause is almost sure to be found in trauma, probably in childhood. That will be the basis for a great deal of the ensuing psychotherapy.

Pain as a dissociative experience

This has been described in an earlier section, but it is worth a second thought, as it is very relevant to this next section.

It means that when someone is in pain, their overall attention is focused on the pain, not on what is going on around them. In other words, they distance themselves from the present to a greater or less degree. The more distance they put between themselves and their surroundings, the greater the dissociation.

This is often an advantage: it prevents outside experiences from interrupting the recognition and, perhaps, the acceptance of the pain. On the other hand, it can be severely disadvantageous, as it diminishes the possibility of distraction from the pain itself and thus may intensify the discomfort.

There are many questions that need to be asked: Does the dissociation mask an important aspect of the pain? Is it the dissociative quality of the pain that interferes with a diagnosis of the cause of the pain? Are emotional factors, and possible dissociative disorder factors, hindering the diagnosis?

There are many possible sources of emotional pain—grief, anger, depression, loss—that can be expressed in a variety of ways.

Emotional pain

A common route of emotional pain is through anxiety. Anxiety attacks are not fun and can create incredible interference in one's life. Such attacks may inhibit performance in the workplace or even jeopardize the job itself; relationship with friends and family may be seriously affected. Often, the person has no idea *why* the attacks occur; they seem to come out of the blue, and they can interfere with almost every aspect of a person's life.

Even more difficult for the client is the merging of anxiety into panic. Again, there is usually no reason why this should happen, but the reality of it is intense.

Often, the course of therapy will turn towards finding the answers to these questions, but that is in the realm of the psychotherapy sessions. In the meantime, people often need tools to keep themselves calm. Hypnosis can sometimes help.

(Lorna has asked about the possibility of using hypnosis to relieve some of the intensity of her anxiety attacks. She is doing well in her therapy sessions, but feels that she needs to learn a new approach for herself.)

Lorna, you've told me about the anxiety and panic that sometimes overwhelms you. Would you like to learn some hypnotic techniques that could ease those episodes? (*Yes*)

Setting the scene

Alright, then, make yourself comfortable and ease into hypnosis to whatever level feels right for you at this time. Signal me when you have reached that level. (*Signals*) Good.

She can sense when she is at that level

Now, knowing that you are safe here in my office, you can allow the tension to ease just a little bit. Not too much—you'll know when it feels best for you. And then, when you have reached that easier awareness, decide whether you would prefer this little technique to be humorous or very straight. (*She will signal you*)

There will almost always be some tension, so remarking on it in a positive way relieves some of the anxiety

Her choice—this is very important

(*If humorous*)
Then you can access your wonderful, rich imagination and clothe that sensation of panic in a costume—a ridiculous costume, whatever you choose it to be. Be sure that the *whole* sensation is clothed in that really ridiculous costume. Yes, that's right, I can see you smiling. It is truly ridiculous, isn't it, that whole panicky sensation? Yes, it is, you're right. Be sure that the *colours* fit the ridiculousness, too—ah, yes, I can see that strikes the right chord. Good.

It can be any kind of costume—an animal, a clown, a wizard, or whatever she chooses

Acknowledge her inventiveness

(*If straight*)
Then you can use your own knowledge
to tell the part of yourself that really gets
overwhelmed with that panic, that you
have a very strong core of yourself, deep
within, that is there to protect you from
danger, and that strong core knows how
to do that. And you can always call on
that strength when you need it most, so
give it a name and use that name any
time, any time, anywhere, whenever you
need to experience that deeper strength.
It's wonderful—do you agree?—to know
that you have that strong, safe part of
yourself, always there for you whenever
panic even begins to show itself.

And you can recognize that early
awareness to your advantage—it's like
having an Early Warning System right
there within you. Yes, that's right.

Now that you know you have the way
to ease and take care of those miserable,
awful panicky feelings, you can rest so
much more comfortably, because it always
feels safer when you know that we have a
solution. Do you agree? (*Nods*) Um-hum.

So come out of your hypnosis now in
your own way, feeling so much more
secure now that you know you have all
the strengths that you need, within you.

**It works well if she has some
sort of image of *strength*—
whatever that might be**

**It is always there, deep within,
so no one can take it away**

**Acknowledging her talents and
strengths**

One more talent—good

***Her* capacity to take care of
herself**

*Notice that these scripts are infinitely malleable—whatever the client chooses—
and offer no specific directions from the therapist as to what the client herself
"should" choose.*

Physical pain

In many ways, physical pain is the easiest pain to relieve through hypnotic
techniques or other altered states of consciousness.

This is because there is a *reason* for the pain; something causes that pain.
When we know that there is a cause, we can direct our attention to that

cause, whatever it might be: injury, infection, allergy, surgery, or physical deterioration such as osteoporosis.

It is also easier because there will be no one telling the client that the pain is "all in their head", which implies that it is imaginary and therefore should be dismissed.

Even in this enlightened day and age, clients come in—often on the verge of tears—and tell me that they have, indeed, been advised that there is no reason for their pain and that they need to "just get over it". It is a situation that invariably makes me furious. "They're just telling me that it's all in my head, aren't they? That it isn't real—I'm just imagining it." Such a scenario is all too frequent when the source of the pain is emotional or has no easily recognized basis.

We can address any one of the several aspects of physical pain—the sensation of the pain itself guides us in that respect. If it is injury, we focus on healing the injury; if it is infection, we can summon up the immune system; if it is surgical, we can look to the future when healing has happened. Hypnotic techniques for these various possibilities usually follow the same thought process, i.e. figure out what is wrong and make it right. Look to the future when the cause has been identified and the pain is healed, or suitable medication is found for problems such as osteoporosis.

We can adapt a rather generalized script to suit these various possibilities. Working with mind–body communication is a crucial part of healing and it is a good way to start. However, it can be much more basic and simple than that. I have vivid memories of lying on the back seat of a car, with my husband and a friend in the front seat, saying to myself, "Healing, Healing, Healing" over and over again to ease the pain of an injured leg. The injury had occurred three days before, and although I had achieved temporary relief with hypnosis, I now had time to do an in-depth session with myself. Along with the mantra, I visualized my leg as comfortable and strong again. By the time we reached London, some six hours later, the pain had left and I knew that recovery would ensue very quickly.

So complexity is not necessary. Keep it simple—just asking the body to do what it has to do in order to help the injured part heal.

Suggest that the client knows, intuitively, the right thing to say, the most useful approach to take. Sometimes the injured person prefers that the therapist vocalizes the hypnosis, so that the client can focus intently on the healing imagery.

Here is one generalized technique, infinitely adaptable to suit any physical pain.

Elaine, you know that there is a reason for this pain and that you are doing whatever the doctor has suggested to help your (*part of the body*) to heal and the (*infection, injury, reaction*) to subside as you get well again.	**Validating the pain: all pain is real, and this pain has a cause** *that has been identified*
Our bodies are truly miraculous in what they can accomplish as they overcome all the physical pain. Just knowing that it *can* happen is an important aspect of the overall situation. You can always keep that in the forefront of your awareness. In fact, you can often watch it happening!	**"Knowing that it *can* happen ..."** **is the essence of healing**
Invite your body to be your teacher, as to how this healing can be achieved. But first and foremost, focus on relieving the pain. As the pain subsides, attending to the other aspects becomes much easier.	**First things first; it is difficult to have a healing image when pain is intense**

Then you may choose to go on with suggestions that are more specific to the situation.

Physiological pain

When I speak about physiological pain, I am thinking of pain caused by some physiological malfunction, such as pain due to a tumour, or a disorder of one of the hormonal glands, or an illness which interrupts body function. "Growing pains" could be an example or pain due to some kind of cancer. It is difficult to differentiate between *physical* pain and *physiological* pain because, of course, they overlap. To clarify the situation, think of pain due to an interruption of a basic physiological process or to physical pain due to an injury. Although this may seem nit-picking, it matters because the approach to one could be less effective if used for the other.

In the following examples, psychotherapy may not be involved as much as it is in other causes of pain, although putting the situation into perspective is always important.

Ellen, you've been telling me about all the tests you've had, indicating that your adrenal glands have been very overactive lately because of a small tumour. It's been causing you considerable discomfort because it is affecting your strength and also because it has been the root of a lot of aches and pains. We've been talking about using hypnosis for the discomfort. Are you interested in beginning that today? (*Yes*)

Identifying the situation

Alright. Then just settle yourself down in a very easy, comfortable position; put a pillow under your knees and make sure that your neck is supported. That's right.

Important to find as much physical comfort as possible

And close your eyes, preparing to go into hypnosis. Good. I see the beginning of a little flutter in your eyelids. Just take your time and go to whatever level feels just right for you today. Nod or show me a finger signal when you have reached that level. (*Nods*)

She herself will know the best level for this experience today

Excellent. Now, in your own way, begin a conversation with that adrenal gland. Talk to it. Say that you know the problem and you also know that the adrenal gland wants to get well; but in the meantime, you need some relief from the discomfort. If you feel like it, reassure that adrenal gland, *again*, that you understand its problem, and you are not angry, but nevertheless, you need some relief. Repetition can sometimes help, almost as if the gland itself has a mind of its own and can be reassured and therefore become more settled.

It is important to allow your logical, cognitive mind to take a rest, while you access the incredibly versatile subconscious mind for this experience

The concept of the body becoming angry is not new; think of an inflamed joint—that also can symbolize anger ("a red, hot, *angry* joint …")

By now, you have an image of that gland, is that right? (*Nods*)

Imagery is the goal

Yes, I thought so. So now you focus on that image and do whatever you need to do to make the image positive and healthy. In your conversation with the gland, reassure it that the doctors are going to (*whatever it is that they are going to do—surgery, radiation, chemotherapy, medication*) so that it can become healthy again and the tumour can shrink or disappear entirely.

Conversing with the body is an integral part of the healing process

Begin to feel more peaceful, and encourage the gland to do so also.

Reassurance

That's right. And from the look in your face, I think that you are more comfortable. Is that right?

And more reassurance

Excellent. So you can continue to have positive conversations with your adrenal gland, as you begin to get well physically through the (*surgery, medication, etc.*).

And even more reassurance

Just stay there quietly in your hypnosis for a little bit longer. Then, when you are ready, begin to come out of your hypnosis gently, reassuring the adrenal gland that you will be in hypnotic contact with it again, very soon.

It is usually helpful to access hypnosis at least twice a day to reinforce the message

Elaborate on this theme in whatever way you wish. Although it seems very far-fetched, remember that in hypnosis, logical judgment is suspended and the perceptive, experiential subconscious takes over.

Organic pain

Generally, organic pain can be thought of as a variable of physiological pain. It can also refer to physical pain, i.e. muscle pain or pain in the various organs of the body (bowel, lungs), or suggest that the pain is deep-seated rather than superficial—superficial, in this regard, meaning literally closer to the surface rather than emotionally shallow.

Barbara, you have been struggling with this great discomfort in your chest for a long time now. The pills your doctor has given you do help a little bit, but the pain is still there, just underneath, and it does interfere with your breathing. Shall we see whether hypnosis could bring a further layer of comfort? (*Yes*)

Acknowledging the help of the pharmaceuticals, but now offering an adjunct to them

Alright. Settle into your hypnosis in your own way, as you have learned how to do. Signal to me when you sense that you are at just the level where you wish to be, in order to learn another tool to relieve the discomfort. (*Signals*)

Something new to learn—always potentially helpful

That's right. Take another moment or two to really make sure, so that you can stop worrying about whether you are at the right level or not. (*Signals again*)

Organizing a receptive mind and body

Good.

Focus, now, on that part of your chest that you instinctively know is the right place to begin. Allow your mind to find the right image for you to contemplate; then, when you sense that you have found that image, begin to breathe softly *right through the image,* as if you were infusing it with clean, pure air. Feel the air passing through your lungs, bringing fresh, healing qualities with it. Now gently, just very gently, breathe. That's right.

It is important that *she* finds the right image, so that this new possibility belongs to *her,* rather than something that has been handed to her

Describing the experience helps to establish it

Continue to breathe in that healing way. You are offering your lungs a safe, simple path toward healing. *Feel* the healing happening. (*She smiles, a little bit*)

Feel—that is, sense—the new possibility; bring in all the sensory qualities

That's very good, Barbara. That's very, very good. You can see how well your subconscious mind—that deep, deep *sub*conscious mind—is helping you to go toward this greater comfort. And your mind and your body are indeed working together, both offering the knowledge that they share.

The *subconscious* mind is the strongest link with the body

Just stay quietly for another few minutes, breathing that healing air through your lungs, bringing relief and comfort. Then take a very deep breath, and bring yourself out of your hypnosis in your own way.

Enjoy the satisfaction of discovery within yourself

Flashback pain

Flashbacks are not the same as what we mean when we say "memories". When we are remembering something, we know that we are in the present, remembering something that happened in the past.

It is quite different to be in the middle of a flashback. It is as if the person is *right back there again*, right in the middle of that terrible situation. They cannot do anything about it, cannot change it, cannot escape it. The full horror of it overwhelms all cognitive sense, and the experiential takes total control.

Flashbacks can occur during sleep and are sometimes misclassified as nightmares. When one has had a nightmare, however, it is recognized as such because it is bizarre, something that never happened and does not connect with reality. Flashbacks connect all too specifically with reality and reopen the wounds—physical and emotional—once again. The sufferer wakens trembling and sweaty, gasping, consumed by anxiety and terror. It is sometimes difficult for them to get back into the present.

To help with this problem, the single most useful thing to do is to establish a code word. And the way to establish this is through hypnosis.

Basic script

Sam, we've been talking about all those flashbacks that you have been having, and how intrusive they are in your life. Often the most difficult part is to get out of them and back into the present.

Establishing the situation

Many people have found that one way to help that along is to have a code word. We've talked about that, and you were interested. Do you feel that this is a good time to establish such a word for you? (*Yes*)

It is important to establish that he is interested in doing that *now*

Good. Then take yourself into hypnosis in your own way, and let me know when you are at a comfortable level to do that. (*Signals*)

Allow yourself to stay quiet and very, very comfortable, just as if you were waiting for something positive to happen. That's right. And while you are in that quiet, comfortable state, ask your wise, deep subconscious to offer you a word that you can use whenever you need to come back into the present, clearly and easily. It can be any word that your subconscious chooses, whether it makes any logical sense or not. Let me know when such a word has come into your mind. (*Wait until he signals*)

Establishing the expectation of a positive outcome

As long as it makes sense to the subconscious it will be useful

Very good. Now, thank your subconscious, and ask it to provide one more word that could also help to re-establish you back into your present presence. Nod when that has happened. (*Nods*)

Always good to have a back-up

Alright. Now, to explore how well that can work, and knowing that you are absolutely safe here in my office, allow yourself to remember—knowing that you are *here* in my office—some scene that you consciously remember that will serve as an example. Let me know when you have found such a scene. (*Signals*)

This is crucial; he must feel safe to be able to do this

Start with a conscious memory, which will be safer

That's right. And while remembering, and feeling the feelings, as if you were right back in the middle of it again, say that code word to yourself, over and over, until the scene fades from your mind. Yes, good. I can see that you are more comfortable.

But encourage realistic awareness

(*You may want to repeat this once or twice more, until you feel sure that he has been able to carry out the suggestion.*)

Very good indeed. Say "thank you" to your subconscious, for helping you in this way. You can now explore those words in your own way, during your own hypnosis time. If you prefer to practice here, in my office, then we can arrange time to do that.

Important to say "thank you"!

(*Often the client will want to do that, until they feel more confident in themselves.*)

Follow-up script

As a follow-up, it can be useful to discuss the memories that come during sleep, i.e. night time flashbacks. I would advise postponing this until he is sure of himself and his ability to bring himself back from a day-time flashback.

So, Sam, you have been very successful in controlling those day-time flashbacks by bringing yourself back into the present. But you are still having interrupted sleep due to night flashbacks. Would you like to establish a way to get some relief from those? (*Yes*)

Clarifying the new challenge

Then go into hypnosis in your own way. That's right. Now, you can establish a code word that you repeat to yourself over and over again *before* falling asleep. It is a different word from the ones that you have been using to control day-time flashbacks. Think of yourself at those other times, in bed and ready to go to sleep. You know that you have been successful in lessening the day-time flashbacks. You can now help yourself to ease the distress from those that occur when you are sleep.

This is the crucial difference between what he has already done and what he is going to do now

Ego-strengthening: he has been before, he can be successful again

As you are just settling into sleep, say your *night-time* code word, over and over. Tell yourself, strongly, that that word is your guardian against the nightmare flashbacks. Repeat the word over and over to yourself, always with the underlying goal of providing a barrier to those interruptions, so that you can enjoy a full, restorative sleep.

This is *prevention* of, rather than coping with, the flashback

And this is the goal

That's right. Very good. You can do it.

Chronic pain

Technically, there is a difference between chronic pain and chronic pain syndrome. Chronic pain refers to pain with an organic (i.e. physical) cause, such as arthritis. Chronic pain *syndrome* refers to pain for which no specific organic cause can be found. That's not to say that there isn't one, but we've not been able to find a way to uncover the root of the problem as yet.

First, let's deal with chronic pain. Obviously, the first task is to ascertain the reason for the pain. Is it injury, inflammation, a tumour? Finding the cause gives a hint as to what kind of hypnotic suggestion might be most helpful.

I've already written about changing the characteristics of the pain. This is an important first step because much of the hypnotic intervention will be to shift the focus of some characteristic of the pain—size, shape, area, edge, temperature, colour—to a different focus, one that is perceived to be more comfortable.

This can be done by direct suggestion or by insinuation.

First script

Doreen, we've been talking about ways to relieve the pain from your injury. The usual things like, hot or cold compresses, support, just haven't been enough. Some medication has helped, but also not enough and besides, it makes you a bit fuzzy and you still have a job to do, injury or no injury.

Setting the scene

We've talked a bit about hypnosis. Are you interested in pursuing that option now? Yes? Very well. Then make yourself comfortable in the reclining chair and let yourself drift seamlessly into whatever level is just right for you this time.

(Scripts for inductions and other general basic hypnotic techniques can be found in many books and journals on clinical hypnosis.)

That's right. When you are ready, tell me something about this pain that you are now experiencing. (*She describes it*) Ah, I think I understand. It is not very big but it is very intense, almost like it's burrowing into you. Is that right? (*Yes*)

Asking her to describe it makes it more real for her, in the sense that she has an image of it

Then let us look at the intensity first. Put it on a scale from 1–10. Where is it? 8? Alright, then imagine a vertical scale in your room, that goes from one to 10. Find out what you have to do to take it from 8 to 7, then 6, and so on. Do that until it gets to a level that is considerably more comfortable.

The 1–10 scale is very useful, and also very adaptable

(Note: people rarely want to take it to one—as if this would be pushing fate too far.)

So that is much more comfortable. Let us leave it at that for today, then, and you can do your own hypnosis at home, at least once a day, to reinforce that change.

Most people would like to work with one or two possible images; more than that becomes too complex

(This is simply an example—you may want to use a shape or a colour or whatever suits you and your client best.)

Second script

If you think that insinuation would be better for your client, you may want to use something like this:

Emily, isn't it wonderful that you have found a way, deep within yourself, to take the edge off that pain that has been bothering you for so long. I wonder what it will turn out to be? It's interesting to know that somewhere, deep inside you, you already know. The mind is truly miraculous and the subconscious even more so.

As you see, this is total insinuation with no suggestion other than "you already know what you need to know".

I look forward to our next meeting, when you can tell me all about it.

Chronic pain syndrome

As we have previously discussed, the title of "syndrome" differentiates between chronic pain that has an organic base and chronic pain—no less disturbing—that seems to have no cause. If anything, chronic pain syndrome is often the more intrusive, simply *because* the reason for it cannot be found.

That reason almost always lies in the past; it may be long past, even back to childhood, or in the more recent past. Both of these—yes, including the more recent past—may be forgotten by the client. Sometimes we forget that which is too painful to remember.

Indeed, I think that this is one of the roots of chronic pain syndrome—a pain whose origin is too painful to remember. Instead, the mind–body connection finds a different way to remember, i.e. through the experience of chronic pain. All too often, as ongoing psychotherapeutic research may yet discover, the pain keeps the cause near the surface, a subliminal subconscious reminder. At a conscious cognitive level, the awareness of the cause of the pain may be ignored; but at the subconscious, perceptual level, it is there and often may be accessed through hypnosis when the client is ready to receive that information.

In these situations, accessing the Mind–Body Communication, Collaboration and Cooperation is always useful. Clients will come in and tell you, "The strangest thing happened—I was just doing my hypnosis and all of a sudden I had this memory …"

But having one or two specific hypnotic techniques is also very useful.

First script

Marlee, we have talked about using hypnosis to relieve some of this pain that has invaded your life. Do you want to start on that today? (*Yes*)

Alright. Then just settle into your hypnosis, as you know how to do, to whatever level seems just right for you this time. Let me know when you are comfortably at that level.

Using the word "comfortably" makes a subliminal suggestion

Knowing that you are safe here in my office, in the comfortable hypnosis chair, you can take your time deciding where you would like to go during this hypnotic time—maybe off to a romantic island, or to a wonderful waterfall, or a special place that is dear to you because of something good in the past.

"Comfortable" again

Implying that there *is* something good in the past

Wherever you have decided to go, take your time and enjoy every moment of the journey, because you are going to a place of healing.

A "place of healing" is another subliminal suggestion

As you get nearer to your destination, you can allow yourself to wonder what it will be like, and to enjoy the positive expectation of comfortableness. You may be wondering whether there will be anyone else there, or how long you are going to stay, or if you will bring something back with you that can remind you of this lovely experience.

More reinforcement of comfort

Imbuing positive expectations

And soon, in your hypnosis time, you can find yourself at your destination, wherever that might be. You may recognize it, or you may wonder if you have been there before. Sometimes a place looks vaguely familiar, but also not quite familiar enough to be able to say, "Oh, I remember now!" You can be very curious about what you will find at that destination.

Again, all these possibilities are positive, something to look forward to; this can block out any potential negativity

Now, I'm going to keep quiet for a little time, so that you can enjoy whatever it is that you are discovering, and how very comfortable you are feeling. You can just allow any small disturbance in that serene awareness to fade away, to dissolve, so that your whole awareness is of comfort.

By reiterating the word "comfort" we can establish a conditioned response—whenever she goes to that same place in a future trance, "comfort" will go there with her

(*After a few minutes*) Marlee, it's nearly time to come back now, so begin to get ready to make that journey, bringing the good feelings with you. You know that you can always revisit that time in the future when you are well again, because that place is within you and you can access it whenever you wish, or need, to do so. Bring back a code word too, to facilitate your travel back to that magical, safe, comfortable place in the future.

Implying that she can and will go back in the future

Here is another possibility.

Second script

Tess, you've been telling me about this pain that seems to have come from nowhere. It was just *there* one day when you went to get up from sitting on the couch. You've said that it was incredibly painful, and although it has eased off a bit, it is still there in the background, just niggling away. You are afraid to move too suddenly, in case it comes back full force again. Is that a reasonable description of the situation? (*Yes*)

Clarifying the situation

And so it is always there, hovering in the back of your mind. Shall we see if we can find a way to dislodge it a bit? (*Yes*)	**Offering a new possibility**
Alright. Then think of your pain, and where it is. Mostly in your back, is that right? (*Nods*)	**Establishing the boundaries**
Then play a little game with yourself, and think of how many phrases you know, and probably use, that have the word "back" in them—my back's to the wall, it gets my back up, back away, I'll get back to you, payback time, everything's all backed up, or others that you also know. Say them over to yourself, very slowly and carefully, and be especially attuned to any response in your body, especially in your back, as you say them.	**Linking the two diverse concepts**
Ah! I see a little frown! Did you have a little niggle of something? (*Yes*)	**If you watch carefully, you can always see a sign**
Then go over your list again, carefully, to discover whether you get that same small message again, and in the same way, or even a different way. (*Give her time to do this*)	**Verifying the connection**
Mm-hum, that's right. Does it seem as if your back is telling you something? (*Nods*) Yes. Then I'm going to be quiet for a few minutes, while you continue that conversation with your back, and we'll see what happens.	**Giving her time to verify the connection**

You will have recognized, by now, that this is a blatant suggestion designed to convert the sensation of pain into a message of some sort. For that reason, you must be particularly careful when using it, or a similar suggestion with other phrases (stand on your own two feet, I put my foot in it, foot-loose and fancy free, I need a leg up)—the list is practically endless and, of course, it differs in various parts of the world, as idioms always do.

You will need to trust your own intuition as to whether your client would respond well to such suggestions. Some will, and in such cases it can be extremely helpful.

You can discuss the implication that the client has identified, and help them apply it in a positive way.

But if you sense that this is not a good approach for your particular client, then follow your instincts and choose another route.

Section II

Stress Disorders

Post-Traumatic Stress Disorder

Post-Traumatic Stress Disorder (PTSD) refers to an emotional and/or psychological response that is higher than the usual level of distress for the presenting situation and is related to events that have happened in the past which have caused sexual, physical and/or emotional trauma to the person who has been injured.

Although depression, phobias, fears and anxiety frequently, if not always, have their origin in past events, they are often not considered as in the same range as PTSD. This section deals specifically with the several types of response that are endemic in "true" PTSD; however, they can also be adapted to suit the other categories listed above.

The language of hypnosis is somewhat different when working with this client population because of the trauma they have experienced. Words and phrases, although understood cognitively, are frequently perceived on an emotional and perceptual level that might bring quite a different perspective. We need to be aware of this and be careful about the way we use those words and phrases.

You may notice that all of the scripts apparently have a positive result. Needless to say, that may not always be the case. Watch for signs of discomfort and, if necessary, gently suggest that perhaps another time might be better for exploring hypnosis. Then you can offer time to discuss the whole idea of hypnosis more carefully. The client may be very good at hypnosis, very comfortable, when using it for other experiences, but may not be ready for exploring this particular type of situation.

Denial

Denial is the first of the several symptoms included in the general category of PTSD-related responses. The person shakes their head—actually or metaphorically—while thinking, "This isn't real; this can't be happening to me." Often people get stuck in this initial response and don't know how to get past it. Hypnotic interventions such as those described below may help break the deadlock. The stage of denial can last for a very long time, overlapping with the other stages to create a kind of emotional chaos.

We can think of the denial as being used to bridge the terrible trauma from the previous, relatively comfortable life to the admission (when they are ready to do so) that it *did* happen—when they can learn how to begin to heal. The client wants, and needs, that bridge.

It is not that there is a "real" version of what happened; it is being able to come to a place where they can acknowledge the experience of it happening.

We also need to remember that the client has been in an altered state during the trauma. There is a difference between that altered state and using the altered state of hypnosis in order to understand how to cope with the memories now. It is important that both client and therapist are comfortable with, and knowledgeable about hypnosis, and that the client already has used and experienced hypnosis and is ready to use it again in this situation.

Strangely enough, the client really wants to be reassured that it did happen—in fact, *must* know that—in order to begin the healing process. The doubting that it happened has occurred, until now, because it has been just too awful to admit. The client is ready to move on.

From time to time, the emotional factor overwhelms. When that happens, "pushing the pause button" offers a time out, as it were, until they are ready to proceed. That may be in the next minute, the next session or the next month. Usually it only takes a minute or so.

First script

Jenny, we have been talking about using hypnosis to relieve some of your distress over the dreadful events of the past. Do you still want to explore those possibilities? Yes, I see you nodding (*or some other signal*), so we can begin.	**Clarifying that she still wants to use hypnosis**

Make yourself very comfortable in hypnosis, going just as deeply into that state as you intuitively know is right for you at this time. Signal to me when you feel you are at the right level. (*Signals*) Thank you. You know that you can change your level of hypnosis at any time in order to feel safer or more comfortable. (*Nods*) Good.

Now, knowing that you are safe in my office and that I am here with you, and will stay with you while you do this, take yourself backwards in time to the day (hour) before those events began to happen. Gradually, let the time in hypnosis time come closer. As that happens, put some distance between you and the events, so that you are watching it from afar, or with an invisible shield between you and the event. Take your time, and let me know when you have reached that state. You can stay calm, knowing that you are simply re-viewing it from a time-distance. (*Signals*) Yes, that's right.

Now, change how time happens, as you are watching this situation evolve. You can just make the time shorter, or longer, depending on whichever is more comfortable for you as you watch. And as the situation unfolds, know that you are there and not there, at the same time, because you are safe in my office, but the event also is very real to you. It is wonderful that we can do and feel both those things at the same time.

She knows where she has to go, and can let you know—this gives her a semblance of power, which she very much needs

It's her hypnosis; she is in control and feeling safe is crucial

Establishing again where she is in reality, and reassuring her that you will not desert her

"Take yourself backwards in time" is an old hypnotic gimmick that always seems to work
Shields are protective, as is some distance between you and what you are watching

Reassuring that she is safe in your office, "re-viewing" it

"Change how time happens" is one of those hypnotic disjunctions that works well in altered states of consciousness; the client will just accept it as normal

"There and not there" is another example, and also very useful

Confirming that it is normal

As you watch, begin to tell yourself that you are watching a *replay* of that terrible time, and because you are watching the replay, so you know that it really happened. You can simply reassure yourself that you are now actually watching the replay, and therefore it really did happen to you and so now you can stop the doubting and the wondering about whether or not it was real; you know that it was real, and because now that you do know that, then the healing can begin.

A replay is very different from the actual experience; one is real, the other is a memory of what was real

But it really did happen—this is an important acknowledgement

You have cleared the barriers and can now move on

Quite often the client will show emotion—tears, huge sighs, or moaning to themselves—and the best thing to do is to let that go on for a few moments, then gently offer encouragement that it is alright now, and that it is nearly time to come out of hypnosis. Bring the client out of hypnosis slowly, again with words of encouragement and validation for the work that they have done.

One of the causes of denial is a sense of guilt—the all-too-common scenario of the victim believing that they somehow caused or invited the trauma. Because that is such a horrendous idea, it is pushed away by the denial that the event even happened.

Second script

Jake, we have talked about using hypnosis to alleviate some of your anxiety about the assault—even wondering whether it had really happened or if you are just making it up in your imagination, manufacturing it for some reason. Are you still interested in discovering what your subconscious mind has to contribute? Yes? Alright, then just settle back in the chair, make yourself comfortable, and go into hypnosis in your own way, however far into hypnosis you instinctively know is the right place where you can explore that concern, at this time.

Usually this conversation takes place before the hypnosis begins; it can normalize the client's concerns. However, we know that clients are in an altered state of consciousness even before the "real" hypnosis begins—indeed, it often begins as soon as they enter the office of a physician or therapist. Therefore we can make use of that time to settle the client and get prepared

Just let me know when you have reached that level of hypnosis. (*Signals*) Thank you. Now, go backwards in time to some time before that event ever happened—perhaps an hour or two before, or a little longer, or a little shorter. See yourself, what you are doing, where you are going—the normal things that make up your day-to-day ideas and experiences. Become very comfortable with those memories of that day. Good.

He gets a chance to go *backwards* in time, so that he can come into the experience, just as it began to happen. Recognizing what happened *before the experience*, makes the next part of the memory credible

In your own time, now—and you know that in hypnosis you can make time go more quickly or more slowly—let yourself begin to recognize the event that is unfolding. See where you are, know what you are doing, feel what you are feeling. Yes, that's right. You can allow yourself to experience what you were experiencing at that time, knowing that you are safe here in my office as you are *re*-experiencing it.

People who are familiar with hypnosis do know this, and feel comfortable with it

Beginning to re-live the event

Repeating the same word is a useful technique in hypnosis, and solidifies the "*experience*"

Clarify, for yourself, that you are really watching what actually happened—seeing, knowing, feeling. If you choose to do so, you can even backtrack the tape, and see it all again and again—as often as you need to do so, in order to believe what you are now allowing yourself to truly perceive.

Validating the memory

This is also a useful technique and allows for doubt to fade and reality to take its place

Take all the time you need, in hypnosis time, to do what you need to do. I'll watch the clock time for you, and let you know.

Another useful gimmick; you can simply say, softly, "Half the clock time is now gone, three-quarters of the clock time is gone ..." etc.

Take a few more moments, now, to make sure that you have answered all the doubts that you may have had about the reality of that event. Then let me know when you are ready to come out of hypnosis, and do so in your own way.

If the client seems to still feel doubt, you can either reiterate the above or if necessary "push the pause button" and save it for the next session. This does work

"Pushing the pause button" fills a dual purpose: it gives the client more time, and it prevents a sense of something still not completed, but that can be accessed later to complete the task.

Hypervigilance

Hypervigilance has its roots, of course, in the need to always be watching one's back. It is one of the most prominent symptoms of PTSD, and one of the most intrusive. It makes trusting almost impossible and interferes with relationships to such an extent that they may be impossible to maintain. It takes great determination on the part of the sufferer to let go of hypervigilance, because the lack of it appears to be an invitation for further trauma. A large part of the psychotherapy for PTSD involves easing this aspect of trauma sequelae. It is difficult for both client and therapist, but is crucial for the return to mental health.

First script

Don, we've talked many times about the intrusion of hypervigilance into your life, and we've also talked about the possible role of hypnosis in easing this factor. Last week, you said that you were interested in exploring this possibility, especially as you have done some hypnosis in the past. Do you still feel that way? (*Yes*) Then let's start in a gentle way, with some easy suggestions that you can begin to use on your own, in your own time. Does that sound like a good idea? (*Yes*)

Setting the scene, making sure that he wants to use hypnosis to help him make changes

Better than storming right in, it offers an easier approach

Alright. Get yourself settled in the reclining chair, then, and ease it back just as far as you wish. Be sure that you at a comfortable angle, and also know that you can change that angle whenever you choose to do so. (*He adjusts the chair*) Good.

He may find that too flat a recline does not feel safe

He's in charge of the recline angle, which is very important. He won't want to be supine

And as we have done some hypnosis before, you know how to take yourself into a safe level for what you are going to do today. Take your time, and let me know when you feel that you have reached that level. (*Signals*)

He knows what the safe level feels like, and what he needs to experience

That's right. Do some breathing exercises for a few minutes, until you know that you are comfortable and that you are in charge of the hypnosis yourself.

Breathing is always good! It helps to stabilize emotions

Being in charge is crucial to relieve the hypervigilance

So, you know how important it is to know that you are in charge of a situation, and you also know how intrusive it can be when something or someone interferes with that situation. And you also know that at times, you need to allow things to evolve, before making a hasty decision. You can monitor carefully—that's often a good thing to do—but you can also allow things to evolve.

Carefully establishing the scene, and the various possible ensuing events, *but* factoring in the idea that at times, allowing a situation to evolve is useful; it might be more interesting and useful than cutting it short

So you can think of a simple situation when it would be useful to allow something to evolve, in order to find out how useful it might be, or to sense the other side of that, which is how intrusive it might be. It takes time and patience to discover those answers. Just let yourself remember something that happened recently, when allowing it to just evolve was, or would have been, a good thing.

Suggesting that he, himself, could think of a *safe* example to explore

Taking time and patience is very important to making a good decision

Have you thought of a situation? Can you tell me just the basics of that situation? Because it is important for you to be able to decipher what part or parts of the situation may be anxiety-provoking for you, or may make you wonder if you are in any kind of potential difficulty. Just give me the general gist of what you are remembering.

The therapist needs to have some idea of what the client is thinking in order to ease the memory into a positive rather than a negative perspective. It is not necessary to have all the details

(The client describes a situation)

Ah, I see. So you were wondering if there is some sort of danger lurking just under the surface, something that you had to watch for, to be vigilant about. Is that right? (*Yes*) Then this is a good example to be working with; you have chosen well.

Bring the hypervigilance right out into the forefront, so that there is no hidden agenda

Supporting the good choice will bolster the positive aspects

It is usually helpful to consider one thing at a time, so choose the first little niggle that comes to you, and easily consider *that one aspect*, remembering that this is a very safe place to do that remembering, and also that you now have the option of *re*-considering. And one thing at a time gives you a chance to keep the main factors in their right order of importance. (*Give him time to do this*)

Part of the problem with hypervigilance is that all the possible dangers are perceived at the same time, thus overwhelming logical thought

And now that you have made this good choice, and had the chance to *re*-consider the situation, you can perhaps perceive it from a slightly different perspective, knowing that you have the wisdom to allow that slightly different possible perspective into that memory, a possibility which can help you in the future as well as in the past.

This is a post-hypnotic suggestion which can ease the intensity of the memory

"In the future as well as in the past ..." is hypnotic language, very useful in such situations; it puts logic into limbo, allowing perception to rule

(*Give him time to conclude this memory and ask him to let you know when he has done so.*)

That was very well done. Now you can understand how helpful it can be, to *re*-consider something from a different perspective. When you are ready, choose another memory from that same situation, in which there may have seemed to be a possible danger, and when you have such an aspect of the memory in mind, just let me know. (*Nods*) Excellent. And now you know that you know how to allow that slightly different perspective to present itself as a possibility, you can do that, as you did a few minutes ago.

"... know that you know ..."— more hypno-speak

I usually keep the "re-considering" to two or, at the most, three mini-experiences in any one hypnotic session. These little scenarios are almost always sufficient to enable the client to start perceiving the episode from a slightly different perspective. You have already helped them to understand that they were over-projecting danger. Let it rest there for a while. Be sure to commend them for the good work, and invite them to come out of hypnosis in their own way. I never debrief the sessions at the time; if the client starts to do so, I usually say, "Let's leave that till next time. You have done very well." Of course, we all have our own opinions on timing and our understanding of our own clients, so use your own common sense—with a good layer of intuition on top of it.

Second script

Harry, you have told me how intrusive the excessive demand for searching out danger has become for you, and you have said that it interferes with your life in many ways. We have also talked about using hypnosis as a means of easing these intrusions. Are you comfortable with beginning that process today? (*Yes*)

Making sure the client is ready

Then settle yourself in the best way that you already know how to do, and take yourself into hypnosis as you did in the sessions we had a few weeks ago. At that time, you were addressing denial. It did seem to be helpful for you when you did that—is that right? (*Yes*) Then that is a good omen, and we can look forward to it being helpful for you again.

If it was helpful before, there is more chance that it will be helpful again

Reassuring him that he is on the right track

You have told me that even going into a nice restaurant is difficult for you. You have to sit in a corner, so that you feel that your back is protected on both sides, and it may be difficult to find a seat where you feel safe. It interrupts what might otherwise have been a pleasant evening. Would it be alright to use that scenario as an example? (*Yes*)

Establishing the scene, and the possible consequence of further problems

In your hypnosis, then—knowing that you are in hypnosis and that you are here in my office—take yourself into a nice restaurant. It is a restaurant where you and your (wife) have visited many times in the past, and enjoyed it. Stay just inside the entrance, recognizing the familiar scene and remembering the pleasant experiences you have had there.

His job to get himself there

He doesn't have to lurch right in

You can enjoy remembering all those past experiences and knowing that this restaurant has always given you good service and a nice feeling.

Establishing good memories and setting the scene for more good memories

Keep remembering the good memories of past experiences in that restaurant. Be sure that you stay just inside the door until you feel very calm and sure about that, and feel confident that this is also going to be a good memory.

Bring the good memories from the past into the present; encourage him to stay with one aspect until it is firmly in place

Let me know when you have that sense of confidence. (*After a few moments, signals "Yes"*)

Wait for the go-ahead

That's good. Now look around and find a nice table where you and (your wife) can sit and enjoy the scene. Look at all those other patrons sitting comfortably at their tables. They know that this is a very nice restaurant and they are relaxed, enjoying the ambience. You can feel that way, too.

He is ready for the next aspect to consider; if you feel he is not yet ready, encourage him to take his time

In other words, if they can be comfortably relaxed, so can he

Focus on getting seated, on looking at the menu, on making your selection. Perhaps you and (your wife) decide to share the appetizer. You feel more comfortable when you are focusing.

More opportunities for focusing, and therefore staying calm

You give your orders to the waitress, then sit back and enjoy a drink or pre-dinner nibbles. Other customers are doing that, so you can also do that. You and (your wife) can chat, or exchange anecdotes and *good* memories. Feel the tension easing from your muscles. Sometimes people, in their imaginations, put the tensions into a safe place, until they choose to look at them again—which may be later that evening or not for months to come. They are kept safe until *you* choose to review them, no matter when that might be. Many times, the tensions eventually just ease away completely, and gently disintegrate. It's up to you.

This whole paragraph is about focusing on the here and now, rather than on scary possibilities that could begin to erode the sense of calm, and of being in control

Putting the feelings in a safe place is a useful gimmick, quick and easy to do at any time and in any place

If you are sensing even the slightest bit of tension, just breathe it away. You know how to do that: find the most comfortable place in your body at this time, breathe all those comfortable feelings in, as you breathe in, then send them right through your body, right to where they are needed, as you breathe out. That's right. It's so easy, and it really works. A few deep breaths, and you are steady again.

Another gimmick—the popular "breathe it in, blow it out" technique that can be used any time and in any place

Using your own judgement, you can take the client right through the meal, through the dessert and through the coffee afterwards! When you have done enough, you can say:

Well, it seems as if dinner is over and it was a very successful experience. What that really means, of course, is that you *can*, as you have just proven to yourself, keep calm and focused as you become re-acquainted with your life. Good for you. We can do another similar hypnosis in a few days, if you wish.

Reinforcing that this is a success story—*his* success story; and if he can do it once, he can do it again, as he gradually begins to integrate the technique into his day-to-day life

Hyperarousal

Hypervigilance and hyperarousal usually go together, one feeding into and the other responding to the situation: the person goes on emotional alert, their biological systems respond in tune; something triggers hyperarousal, and the mind looks around for danger. As I have said hundreds of times, in workshops and to clients, we are never disconnected at the neck.

First script

Jerry, we talked last time about some major concerns of yours, and especially about your emotional response when it had been triggered in some way. You felt as if your whole body was reacting to that trigger—whatever it was that was the focus of attention at that time—so much so that your thoughts were quite illogical and intrusive. You said that you were never able to sort out those responses.

Making sure the issue is clear and he is aware of the hyperarousal for what it is

We talked about the possibility that some hypnosis might offer a new venue, as it were, to look at this from a brand new perspective, a different angle. Do you still want to do that? (*Yes*) Then let's explore, and see what we find.

Reinforcing that this is just another perspective, rather than something to be wary of

You've done hypnosis in the past, so you know what to do. You can just make yourself comfortable and go into hypnosis in your own way, as far as you just know, intuitively, is the right level at this time. Let me know what you have reached that level. (*In time, he nods or signals*) Good.

Getting settled

Let's start with something very simple and familiar, shall we? Think about (your wife) coming home from a short trip away. You go to meet her, and find yourself a little bit agitated as you wait for her, even though you know that she is fine. Allow yourself to feel those feelings, Jerry; you can describe them to yourself or, if you wish, out loud.

Choose a familiar scenario to add to the settled feeling

There are both advantages and disadvantages to his speaking out loud. Depend on your instincts

Now, feeling those feelings, also be aware of how your body is responding to them. Always remember that we are never disconnected at the neck, and our minds and our bodies both respond to situations, simultaneously. You are aware of the *emotional* part—the feelings of a little tension or even a little anxiety; now also be aware of how your *body* is feeling. Is it tense also? (*After a moment, "Yes"*)

Making the mind–body connection more specific

It's good that you can recognize that. Keep on paying attention to your body's responses. Are you aware of some other ways in which your body is telling you that it is upset or concerned also?

Encouraging his discovery

There are almost always other symptoms

At this point, he may tell you that his heart is beginning to hammer, or his hands feel damp, or that he can't seem to take a deep breath in. Reassure him that he is doing a good job of recognizing these symptoms.

42

Yes, you can understand how your mind and body are both responding, can't you? Now, in your imagination, you see (your wife) coming towards you, and you feel an immediate emotional relief. Yes, that feels better, doesn't it? (*Yes*)

More reassurance

Re-connecting the mind–body from the opposite standpoint

Just take your time, in hypnosis time, now, and begin to feel better in every way. Tell me when you reach that comfortable state. (*After a few moments, he nods*)

Excellent. You have done a very good job, Jerry, experiencing and understanding how mind and body always go together. It helps to understand that, as we both know; so now you can comfortably come out of hypnosis in your own way, knowing that you have learned, or even re-learned, something very important today.

Reaffirming that he has, indeed, learned from the experience

Second script

This script often fits nicely into the next session, or soon after, so that it is an easy continuation of his learning curve. Of course, it can be used singly, also—whatever seems appropriate.

Well, Jerry, after your excellent hypnosis session the other day, are you interested in learning another technique for reducing the physiological response and also, at the same time, the emotional response to the triggers? (*Yes*)

Reassuring and, at the same time, encouraging further work

I thought that you might be. So settle in, then, and reach that level of hypnosis that you know is right for you at this time.

Now, when you are ready, imagine being in a situation that arouses all those physical responses. You know that you are here in my office, and that (I'm a physician), so you can feel very safe, in another part of your awareness, while you are doing this useful hypnotic exercise.

He can choose his own situation and will do so, according to his sense of what is appropriate for him at this time

I see that your breathing is changing a little bit, so I gather that you are imagining, or remembering, some worrisome scenario. Is that right? (*Yes*) I thought so, and I assure you that I will watch you carefully, and that you are safe, experiencing those messages that your body is sending you.

Begin with the breathing; it's an obvious symptom and it is also linked to heart rate, which will be next

Watch your client carefully, noticing the pulse in the neck, the rate of breathing, muscle tension in the body, and other signs of agitation. When you sense that he is becoming overwhelmed, then say:

Hold it! That's right, just hold it right there! Now, start reversing those symptoms, and begin with the breathing. Just focus on your breathing, and bring it back into an easy, comfortable, natural rate. Take your time.

Putting the experience on hold for a moment; the client will always respond by doing just that—and stay in a sort of limbo for a few seconds

You may choose to breathe with him, slowing your own breathing down as he begins to slow his. As he returns to a reasonable rate, you can say:

Very good. Now, attend to your heart rate, which will already have settled somewhat because breathing and heart rate are linked physiologically. Um-hum, that's right. When you have settled into a comfortable, normal heart rate for you, choose the next symptom: perhaps your hands are wet, or your stomach is in a knot. Just reverse that symptom, too, and continue to do the same thing with all those physical awarenesses, until you know that you are back to normal. You can take a deep breath to let me know that, too.

Physiologically true, so it is a wise reassurance to give He keeps his own pace and routine as he continues to reverse the symptoms

Sometimes, you may choose to do the whole thing again, which is useful as long as the client agrees. Reassure him that he did it very well, and his ability to do it in other circumstances can be reinforced by doing it again now.

Jerry, you have done an excellent job today. During the next few weeks, you can practice reversing the symptoms any time that you recognize them, and soon you will find that you can do it spontaneously without having to even think about it. As that happens, you will have reached another level of healing.

As he is still in hypnosis, this is a post-hypnotic suggestion
Healing is the goal

Lack of trust

Lack of trust is one of the most basic and negative qualities of Post-Traumatic Stress Disorder. That is not hard to understand, because the "trauma" in PTSD was unfair insofar as there was nothing the victim could have done which would or could have stopped it.

Furthermore, that negativity is often emotionally transferred in such a way as to make the victim believe that they were, at least in some way, responsible for it. The lack of trust therefore extends to the sufferer too, which adds to the unfairness of it all. This last point is one of the reasons—probably the main reason—why lack of trust *in oneself* is the first and most crucial aspect to address. The lurking worry of "If only I had ..." needs to be assessed.

You may recognize in these scripts that hypnotic suggestions are frequently used to urge the process forward. The following script has several of these, suggesting that "deep inside (herself), she *knows* ..." Basically, this is enhancing her sense of self-worth, an essential component of trust in oneself.

First script

Diane, we have spoken several times about how hard it is for you to trust anybody or anything—we even had a little laugh when you said you didn't even trust your cat. Do you think that you are ready now, to start to address that basic quality? (*Yes*)

Opening up the topic; making a very small joke that you have shared before, to settle her

Good. And we have talked about starting this process by using hypnosis. Are you still alright with that idea? (*Yes*)

Checking this out also

Fine. Then take yourself into hypnosis, as you know how to do, and settle at a comfortable level—one where you know that you know where you are and what you are doing but nevertheless have a protective hypnotic wall around you. Does that sound reasonable? (*Yes*)

She needs to find her own level of hypnosis, both because she can make the choice herself, and is therefore in charge, and because she can provide the safety wall

You do that, then, and tell me when you are ready.

(*Signals*) Alright. I know that you have told me, on more than one occasion, that there were occasions when people didn't believe you, even though *you* knew that you were telling the truth. Think of such an instance. You don't have to tell me about it, although you can if you wish. Are you thinking of such a time? (*Yes*)

Reminding her that she already has this knowledge about herself

She may or may not choose to tell you; telling is dangerous

Good. Now, go very, very, *very* deep inside yourself, as one can do in hypnosis, until you reach the place that tells you how you *know* that you are right in what you are saying. Nod when you deeply, truly, *know* that. (*Nods*)

Whether this statement is "real" or not doesn't matter; this is "hypno-logic", i.e. perception

That's excellent. Now, find out what it is, deep inside you, that allows you—even *insists*—that you truly know and believe that you are right. Signal when you know. (*Signals*) Yes, that's right. You truly, deeply *know*, and *believe*, that you are right in what you are saying and thinking. Have you reached that place yet? (*Nods*)

More hypno-logic; again, we are dealing with how she perceives herself and/or the situation

Reaffirming

I'm very glad for you, because now you truly, deeply know that there is one person on this earth that you can trust, and that person is you, yourself. That is truly a marvelous thing to know, and to believe, and to have as a certainty within you.

The point of the whole exercise: "you can believe in yourself"

Yes, it is. Just rest with that wonderful knowledge for a few minutes—as long as you like in hypnosis time, a few minutes by clock time. I'll watch the clock time for you. (*Advise her as time passes, for about thirty seconds*)

You have made a wonderful decision—to believe in your *self* and therefore to trust in yourself. That means that you can stop second-guessing everything you do, every decision you make. If you want to make sure that it is the right decision, you can just take a few seconds, go very deep within yourself, and check it out. Imagine it being so easy!

"Your *self*" and "yourself" are deliberate, and meaningful for enhancing self-worth

Strengthening the decision, the perception

And more hypno-logic—very, very useful

And I know that you will always make *very* sure about those decisions, because you do know that you can trust yourself. And if, from time to time, you have that slightly uneasy sense that makes you want to review the decision again, you know that you can do that, too, trusting yourself to check it out.

This wonderful capability is going to stay with you, strengthening the inner trust

Take a few moments, now, to really sense what has happened within you. You have discovered that you can indeed trust yourself; and knowing that, that it will help you to decide *when* and *why* and *if* you should trust somebody else. Just stay with that thought for another few moments, and then bring yourself out of hypnosis in your own way.

Preparation for beginning to trust other people, when they deserve to be trusted

Second script

You and your client are also engaging in the psychotherapeutic process, as well as hypnosis. That part of the interaction with the client is the time for putting their new understanding and recognitions on the table, so that together you can evaluate them. With Diane, you would want to know more about the qualities that she discovered within herself, now that she has identified them, and how those recognitions are affecting her day-to-day life.

Diane, you have been exploring your own trust in yourself for some time. Do you feel that you are ready now, to take the next step, and discover what it may be like to trust others? (*Yes*)

Defining the task

Just prepare yourself, then; make sure that you are very comfortable, and ready to move on to the next stage. Nod when you have reached that point. (*Nods*)

She must feel ready herself

Good. Now, do a quick scan of your life and find *one* person, just *one*, that you just instinctively, intuitively, knew how to trust. It can be someone from any time in your life, it doesn't matter when.

Only one person is needed for this part of the healing to begin

(*If your client chooses you, thank them, say how honoured you are, and suggest that, for the purposes of this exercise it would be better to choose someone else. Usually, but not always, they will choose someone from either childhood or from the very recent past, perhaps a new liaison. Either can have pitfalls, so monitor carefully.*)

Good. You have already recognized some qualities that lead you to believe that this person is, or was, trustworthy and safe. Now check out for yourself just what those very special qualities are. And it is important to look at those qualities from a distance, as if you were watching a movie or TV.

Intuition is very important, but so is checking it out

"Distance" is also important

Take your time, to be sure that you are sure. Are you sure that you have identified those excellent, important qualities? (*Nods*) Good.

Now comes the really interesting part! You remember that you were able to recognize qualities within yourself that made you trustworthy. Find out now whether those same qualities are part of *this* person's real character.

This is a crucial aspect of the exercise; it reinforces her belief in herself, and prepares for a belief in the person she has chosen, *if the same qualities are there*

If they are, then you have discovered yet another important factor in the trusting relationship; if they are *not,* then you have discovered that you can recognize safe, trustworthy qualities when you see them, and that is a very important talent to have.

Either way, she wins

We still have some interesting work to do regarding trust; but perhaps this will be a good time to stop today, so that you can put it all into perspective.

Preparing for next time and also giving her some "homework"

When you are ready, bring yourself out of hypnosis in your own way.

Third script

Diane, now you have had a couple of weeks to think about the work we've done together recently. I think that you have done very well. What do you think? (*Some comments regarding her own progress*)

Getting ready for the next step

It is important that *she* has some comments

Yes, those are good comments. Are you ready to go on to the next step? (*Yes*) Good. Then settle into hypnosis in your own way, as you know that you can do very well. Let me know when you have reached a very comfortable level. (*Signals*) Good.

Making the commitment to proceed

Last time, in your hypnosis, you found one person with whom you knew you could feel a sense of trust. And you were able to utilize that realization in a positive way.

Re-establishing the scenario, and emphasizing the importance of a level of trust

49

Today, you can explore a little further. In your own way, seek out someone whom you know, but do not *really* know, and explore your real feelings towards that person, especially with regard to trust. Just recognize your own innate sense of whether that person deserves your deep trust. These thoughts are just within you, so you can make them as clear as you wish, because nobody else has to know them.

On to the next step—the next level of complexity

The innate sense of trust in herself is crucial

It is private, one's own feelings or gut reaction

Just signal when you know what you know. (*Nods*)

Now, if you know that you know that you can really trust that person, then you can have that sense of security. Let me know if you do have that sense of security.

There has to be that sense of certainty in herself

If "*no*": Aha! You recognized that lack of real assurance, deep within you. Good for you. Now you can do the very same exploration again, and see what else can happen.

Something not quite right here

If "*yes*": Aha! So now you know that you can recognize that quality in someone, that deep sense of trustworthiness. That is a special talent, to be able to recognize that, and you have that very special talent.

Something reassuringly right here

At this point, if the answer was "no", one can encourage the client to again choose someone else, and see what happens (and this could repeat several times—I usually let it happen a maximum of three times before saying, "You are doing an excellent job of recognizing your own capability to sense trustworthiness, or the lack of it. Let's finish for today, and you can rest comfortably, knowing that you know how to recognize those important factors."

On the other hand, if the client feels that they have indeed sensed a level of trustworthiness, then you can go on as follows.

So now that you know that you have that very special talent, bring into your present awareness some person whom you do know, perhaps whom you have known for a very long time and that you like, and allow yourself to discover what there is to discover, about that person. You can sense whether or not to trust him or her, and that will add a new dimension to your relationship.

And now the next step—to apply that new knowledge, which in turn will bring a kind of reassurance that the client can have *self*-trust, which is an essential ingredient in developing trusting relationships

Let yourself be comfortable with your new awareness, and, with that increasing ability to recognize what you need to recognize in order to be safe, you can indeed feel safer.

Flashbacks

There is a major difference between memory and flashbacks. When we are remembering something, we know that we are in the present recalling something that happened in the past. However, when someone is having a flashback, they are *right back in that situation again* with all its horrors—its sights, smells, sounds, pain and terror. As always, when working with dissociative experiences, we must be careful to avoid flipping the client right back into the same terrifying state.

Flashbacks sometimes occur during sleep and may be mistaken for nightmares; the same criteria apply, however, because night flashbacks are from real situations, as they were experienced, and not something that the subconscious weaves together to create a bad dream. Usually the obvious fear experienced by the person having the flashback can relate directly to the fact that it is a flashback and not a dream or nightmare.

Personally, when I am working with flashback situations I do not deliberately use a hypnotic state, with the usual induction and settling in. The experiences of flashbacks are so dreadful that it seems to me that it causes needless distress to do so. Instead, I make use of the altered state of consciousness that the client is already experiencing when in a flashback or even when telling me about it. Therefore, there can be several different scenarios. I usually speak as if the client *were* in a "regular" hypnosis—that is, I don't expect verbal responses, although they sometimes happen. (But they sometimes happen in specific hypnosis, too!)

It is often important—especially with those who have experienced significant trauma—to discuss with the clients ways of keeping themselves safe. That includes keeping yourself safe in the hypnotic milieu. Techniques may include putting up an invisible wall, wrapping a protective cloak around yourself, watching from a distance as if in a theatre, and other similar techniques.

First script

Jason, you have told me something about the flashback that you had yesterday. It seemed to have been particularly nasty. Let's find a way to minimize its impact on you, shall we? (*Yes*)

A positive goal

Alright. You know how important it is for you to feel safe when you are describing these experiences to me, so do whatever you need to do to make yourself feel safe now. Let me know when you are feeling comfortable enough to tell me about it.

Reassuring that he can help himself to feel safe

(*After sufficient time has passed*) Yes, that's right, Jason. You look as if you are more settled and feeling somewhat safer; that sense of feeling somewhat safer is often the case when you know that you are here in my office—is that right? (*Nods*) That's good. Take a few moments to *know* that you are safe, here in my office. (*Appears to settle, sighs*)

Positive feedback, although you may need to embellish a bit

And are you feeling protected, now, also? (*Nods*) That's good.

Feeling safe and feeling protected may not "feel" quite the same

Begin to tell me, just in general terms, what the flashback was about. For example, where were you, at the time, in the flashback, and where were you in real time?

Stating the obvious discrepancy in the experience of time

The client begins to describe the situation. Below, I am describing a common sort of scenario; you will need to adapt it to suit you and your client's needs.

So you are looking out the window of the train, and see the huge curve coming up, too fast—very, very fast. Now begin to breathe, in the way that you know how to do, before you begin to tell me any more about that experience. Breathe slowly and steadily, as you know how to do. That's right.

Whatever the situation might be, the emphasis on controlled breathing is always important, as it is one of the body experiences in which we can have some control

Often it helps to breathe <u>with</u> the client, in the same rhythm, loud enough so that they hear you echoing their breathing; then as you begin to modify yours, perhaps a little more slowly, so does the client. It is a spontaneous response.

That's right, Jason, just breathe. You can settle yourself down a little bit, that way, even though you see the sharp curve that is coming up so quickly. You may even have time to find the emergency exit, or decide which window you may break if you need to do that. You can have greater sense of control, just from focusing on your breathing.

Offering some possible solutions

That's right. Now, Jason—*NOW*, Jason— look at me. Look at me and tell me where you are. Look right at me, and tell me just where you are right now. Feel your feet on the floor; feel the arms of the chair you are sitting in. It is different from the seat in the train, isn't it? You can recognize all those differences, Jason. Tell me about the place where you are, right *NOW*.

It is often important to speak in a very loud, firm voice, to bring his attention back to the here and now

Yes, that's right, you are here in my office. Just look at me, and then look around you and you will see the familiar furniture, the pictures on the walls, the mat on the floor. Feel the arms of the chair again, with your hands. That's right.

Reassuring and reaffirming

You can use the same techniques if someone goes into a spontaneous flashback and you are there. "Look at me; tell me who I am; you know me; what is your name; tell me your name; look down at the floor/sidewalk/grass/rug and tell me what you see; breathe; breathe again, pay attention to your own breathing ..." etc.

Jason, you handled that very well. Now you know that you can, indeed, minimize the miserable intrusion of these flashbacks into your everyday life. Of course, it takes time and practice, but you *can* do it— you've just proven that you *can* do it. As you practice these techniques more and more, you can gain more and more self-assurance, and a re-awakening of your own power.

Essentially, this is a post-hypnotic suggestion, as he is in an altered state of consciousness and therefore more receptive

Second script

The script below should probably be postponed until the client has had considerable success in recognizing flashbacks in retrospect, and is ready to be more proactive in dealing with them.

Jason, you have been doing good work in coping with your flashbacks in retrospect. Are you ready, now, to work on prevention, instead of re-experiencing these miserable situations? (*Yes*)

Recognizing past effort, being sure that he is ready to move to the next step

Alright; then tell me whether you think it could be helpful, if I suggest a trigger word while you are here in my office, where you know that you have my support should you need it. Are you comfortable with that? (*Yes*) Please be very sure that you know that we can push the pause button at any time, and not release it until you choose to do so. Do you really *know* that you can do that? (*Yes*) Then settle yourself in the chair and tell me or signal to me when you are ready.

This gives him some warning that his subconscious will recognize as such, and begin preparing

An easy and important safety factor

(*After a short time, he signals*) Thank you. Remember, keep your eyes open so that you really know where you are. You will also need to hear my voice, so tell me if I speak too softly. (*Nods*) And you know that we can stop the session any time you choose. Will you tell me or signal me, if you need to stop the session? (*Yes*) Alright.

Very important that he keeps his eyes open. Stop and/or backtrack if the eyes close

Remember that the following is just a suggestion of what you might do at this time to help your client deal with flashbacks. Be sure that <u>you</u> are sure that both of you are ready to undertake this next stage.

Jason, LOOK OUT! IT'S COMING! LOOK OUT, JASON!

A very common trigger

Jason begins to react in some way—looks around desperately, breathing starts to become rapid, eyes open wider, etc. You recognize that he is beginning to re-live some experience, triggered by your phrases. Allow this to happen for a few minutes, not more than two or three at the most, and then begin to bring him back from the evolving flashback situation.

Jason, now look at me. Just look at me. Tell me where you are. Where are you right now, Jason? Look around at the room we are in; what room are you in, Jason? Look at the rug on the floor. Feel your feet on the floor. Touch the arm of the chair. Tell me who I am.

Beginning the re-alerting into the present

You keep on in this manner until he has reoriented himself back into your office.

Jason, you did that very well indeed. You can be proud of yourself. See? You are learning to unlearn all those intrusive triggers and deal with them in a logical fashion by recognizing who you are, where you are, who is with you, what you are doing, and other similar feelings and awarenesses. Good work!

"Learning to unlearn ..." is an hypnotic suggestion

Sleep flashbacks

Flashbacks that occur during sleep are often misinterpreted as nightmares. It takes time and skill to differentiate the two, but the first and most important factor is whether or not the so-called nightmare made sense; that is, if it seemed to be a very real experience, rather than the illogical, disconnected and partial events that indicate a nightmare.

When you are quite sure that your client is experiencing sleep flashbacks, you may want to use one of the following patterns. You can either suggest a familiar hypnotic induction, or simply rely on them to go into hypnosis comfortably, in the usual way.

First script

Maureen, you have told me several times
about the disturbing events that happen
during the night, when you are asleep,
that seem to be nightmares and yet are
too clear and real, more like a re-living of
an actual experience—*your* real experience
of that terrible accident. You've said that
it seems as if you are right back in that
dangerous and frightening place and
time, and you can remember it all too
clearly when you wake up. Is that right?
(*Yes*)

Clearly identifying the situation

We have talked about these intrusions
as possibly being flashbacks, rather than
nightmares. Does that still seem to be the
case? (*Yes*)

**More clarification—it is very
important to do this**

Then I have a suggestion. Perhaps one or
two hypnosis sessions might be useful,
with a positive post-hypnotic suggestion.
Would you like to explore that possibility?
(*Yes*) Good. As you know, hypnosis brings
its own response which may be different
for different people. That's normal. It
seems like a good idea; it is safe, you are
here in my office with me, and it could be
helpful.

**Reassuring that this is to be a
suggestion to the subconscious**

Settle yourself in, then, and take yourself
into hypnosis in your own way. Take your
time—we have lots of time. Signal to me
when you feel that you are at the right
level. (*In a few moments, signals*)

**Time is always distorted in
hypnosis, so "lots of time" can
be taken at face value**

Now, you can just imagine yourself in your own home, getting ready to go to bed. It's night time, you are tired, you've had a busy day and you're sleepy. Take yourself through all your usual bedtime routines. You can enjoy doing that, because you know that you are going to have a good night's sleep and will awaken in the morning refreshed and ready to start the day. That's right, just settle into that time and space.

Setting the scene more clearly and specifically, using the very ordinary bedtime routines to bring even more relaxation

Before you go to sleep, it's nice to do some self-hypnosis, just a short session, as you know how to do. Yes, I can see that you are doing that very well. In your self-hypnosis, re-affirm that you will have a very serene, comfortable sleep, right through the night. Any dreams you may have are pleasant, and you can enjoy them because in your dreams, you are experiencing happy times. You know that you are safe in your own home.

This makes the client even more active—a participant rather than in the audience

This is the crucial post-hypnotic suggestion

An important statement—he or she is *safe in (her) own home*

If the client has a spouse or partner, the therapist can add a few words about that extra degree of safety, if appropriate. If that is questionable, then plan how you might discuss such a situation.

Take yourself right through the night, safely and comfortably, knowing that you can have that safe, comfortable sleep each and every night, because that is what is right for you.

The security lasts all night, every night

Now, still in your hypnosis, waken in the morning feeling refreshed and ready to start the new day.

And is still there in the morning

You can always have that refreshing, safe, restoring sleep, and you can use your own hypnosis to make that sleep time even more comfortable.

Now, in your own way and your own time, bring yourself out of hypnosis and back into my office. That's right.

Second script

Not everyone can make the following exercise work for them, but it's a very good one when that does happen. Some people have the capacity to know when they are asleep—the so-called "lucid dreaming". For anyone with this capacity, the following script can be very helpful. It is not for everyone, however; and it is complex, deliberately so, in order to create a confusion. Hypnosis is about disjunctions, and there are times when the deliberate use of hypnotic techniques to create a kind of confusion can result in the mind finding its own explanation, whether or not it makes sense rationally.

Barry, we have talked in the past about your capacity to know when you are sleeping—a talent that only a few people have, yet one that apparently can be acquired and utilized. This is very much like a lucid dream, one in which you know both that you are asleep and also that you are dreaming. The ability to do this can be cultivated in someone who knows that he has that capacity but has never deliberately used it. Perhaps it can be useful for you, when you experience your night flashbacks. Does that make sense to you? (*Yes*)

Defining the experience of lucid dreaming

Implying that he has that capacity and could learn to use it

Alright, then, let's see how this could work when we bring hypnosis into the mix also. That would make a powerful mixture—do you agree? (*Yes*)

Layering hypnosis on top of lucid dreaming

Then let us explore the possibility. Take yourself into hypnosis, to a deeper level than usual, and let me know when you know that you have reached that level. (*Signals*) Thank you.

Presenting this as a challenge

Now, *in your hypnosis,* perceive yourself as if you were sleeping, in that special wide-awake sleep that you can recognize. Let me know when you have reached that place. (*Signals*)

Setting the scene

Good. Now, *transfer that awareness* into a recognition that you are having a sleep-flashback, and then respond as you would if you were just dreaming but wide awake.

This is where it becomes a new skill, with the implied suggestion that he can do it

In other words, you can realize that you are really asleep and dreaming, although it is as if you are wide awake. But knowing that you are actually experiencing a flashback, you can bring yourself *out* of that strange experience by waking up.

It becomes more cognitively confusing, which is useful when including hypnosis

So now it is time to bring yourself out of both the flashback lucid dream, and also of the hypnosis. Take your time, and come back comfortably.

Re-establishing cognitive thought

As I have said, this is not a technique for everybody: it is challenging and it also requires the capacity for lucid dreaming, and then the subconscious recognition and ability to unite those components. But it is wonderful when it works, giving clients the knowledge that they have a special ability to be able to control those aspects of PTSD which intrude so violently into their lives.

Other sleep disorders

There are other sleep disorders that those with PTSD experience: various types of insomnia, interrupted sleep, difficulty getting to and maintaining sleep, and fear of something bad happening while they are asleep. At times, very simple hypnotic techniques can allay many of these problems.

First script: The blackboard technique

Jill, we talked for a little while last time about your concern that you are just not getting enough sleep. I suggested that some simple hypnotic techniques might perhaps be helpful. Now, are you still interested in pursuing that? (*Yes*)

Making sure that she is still interested

Alright. Then let's start with the simplest of all sleep-inducing techniques. It is an old technique that I have used many times, and from what I have been told, it seems to be effective for most of the people who explore it. If this one turns out to be less helpful for you than we wish it to be, I do have others up my sleeve, so you can stop being discouraged. Shall we begin? (*Yes*)

Reassurance, that it is a simple and useful technique

Everybody has their own feelings about what may be useful

Then take yourself into hypnosis in your own way, and let me know when you feel that you would like to learn this simple, easy-to-use program. (*In a few moments, she signals*)

Very good. Now, take yourself, in your own way, to a time when you are getting ready to go to bed. You have washed and brushed your teeth, and made your usual bedtime preparations. And you are looking forward to a very comfortable, refreshing sleep, so you want sleep to come easily and quickly. You get into bed, and snuggle down into the pillow, and bring the soft blankets up to where you like them.

Setting the scene more specifically

Imagine this, in your mind's eye. There is a blackboard; you are holding a piece of chalk in one hand and a blackboard eraser in the other. Have you got that? (*Yes*) Good.

Here is where it gets interesting, because there is something new in the scene

Now, in the middle of the blackboard, put the numeral "1". You can look at it, and admire it—the straight line, or with a little hook on top, or the little hat and shoes that the numeral may seem to be wearing. Or maybe you have made a Roman numeral—whatever seems to suit you best.

Something specific for you to do in your hypnosis

After admiring it, you erase it; and then in the upper corner of the blackboard, you print the word "sleep". You look at it, and admire it, and erase it.

More specific requirements—all the more interesting as you proceed

In the middle of the blackboard, you print the numeral "2". I wonder how you'll fashion the numeral "2"? Will it have nice curves in it? Have you chosen to use a Roman numeral? Will your numeral "2" have a sort of flat step along the bottom? Do it in your own, special way, because it is *your* numeral "2".

Continuing with the stage setting

You look at it for a few moments, then admire it, and erase it.

It's just the right thing to do

In the upper corner of the blackboard, you print the word, "sleep". Then you admire it, and erase it.

More repetition: *interesting!*

In the middle of the blackboard, you put the numeral "3". There are several ways to form the numeral "3": you can have two half-circles—sometimes with the top one smaller than the bottom one; or you could have a diagonal line through the middle of the "3"; or perhaps you have some other special, very personal way of writing the numeral "3"; and of course, there is always the possibility that you might like to use Roman numerals.

Continuing in the same pattern—becoming routine, but at the same time, intriguing

You look fondly at your numeral "3", admire it, and erase it; and in the top corner of the blackboard, you print the word "*sle-ee-e-p*", paying particular attention to the "*ee-e-eee-e-s*". You admire it, and erase it.

**"Where is this going?" one might be wondering
As you say this, change your tone of voice to reflect the vocal quality: "*sle-ee-e-p*", "*ee-e-eee-e-s*"**

In the middle of the blackboard, you write the numeral "4"… and you continue in this way, the numeral and then the word "slee-ee-ep", until you wake up in the morning.

Aha! So there is a purpose, after all. Where will it lead? Yes, very intriguing, indeed

And when you wake up, you can be very
surprised when you remember what the   **What will the surprise be?**
last number that you wrote had been.

I have used, and taught, this technique many, many times and it almost always
proves to be useful. I have had people complain that they only managed to count
to "1", and they feel cheated. On the other hand, one man said to me that he had
counted up to 250, at which time he became annoyed and gave up! Applying the
tonal quality to "sleep" and the letter "e" is an implicit invitation to go to sleep
easily.

N.B. This script is very similar to one in *Creative Scripts for Hypnotherapy.*

Second script: Wading into sleep

(Advice: Be very sure that your client has no fear of the water before you
suggest this particular script.)

Well, Jan, you said that you would be
back to learn some hypnosis for getting to
sleep, and here you are. Do you feel ready
to explore that today? (*Yes*)

Good. Then let yourself ease into a very   **If the client is not familiar with**
comfortable level of hypnosis—one that   **hypnosis, then that previous**
just suits you perfectly right now—and   **experience has to happen first**
we can begin. Nod when you feel you are
at the right level. (*Nods*)

Yes, you look very comfortable, and as if   **Feeling safe is very important**
you feel safe. Is that right? (*Yes*)

You enjoy being near the water, isn't that
right? (*Yes*) So you can imagine yourself   **Setting the scene**
at a lovely beach. It may be one that you
know well, and have often visited, or it
might be one that you conjure up in your
imagination. The important thing is that it
feels just the right place, right now. Let me
know when you are there. (*Signals*) Thank
you.

Now, stroll down the beach, until you find a spot that appeals to you, and seems to be just the right spot to wade into the water. You can go slowly, and enjoy the feeling of the cool water on your skin, as it is quite a warm day, isn't it? (*Yes*)

Just enjoy easing yourself into the water, in your own time, in your own way. As you go further and further, deeper and deeper into the water, you enjoy the lovely, soothing sensation of the water beginning to surround your body, first your feet, then your legs, your hips and your abdomen, your waist—all the way up until you are just as deeply into the water as you wish to go, in deeply enough so that you can just float so *very*, very comfortably in the water.

Look up at the blue sky, the wispy clouds passing by. Oh, what a lovely sight! You can close your eyes and yet still see those beautiful, soft clouds in that wonderful blue sky.

The soft sensation of the gentle wave-like motion of the water is so soothing, that it almost feels as if you could drift off into sleep, and yet still stay floating, safely and securely held up by the water. Mmmm. So gentle and soft, so safe and comfortable. You may even hear the sound of gentle waves on the beach, or hear the shimmery whispering of the leaves in the trees.

You can stay there as long as you wish, in hypnosis time. I can watch the clock time for you, and let you know when the time nears for you to bring yourself back from the beach—but for now, you can continue to enjoy that delightful drifting, the easy, wavy motion that soothes and comforts. Mmmmm.

She needs to feel like a participant, not an observer

Focusing on the soothing sensation

Enjoying the view as well as the physical experience (always use as many perceptions as possible)

Safely and securely—very, very important so it needs to be stressed

"Clock time" and "hypnosis time" are very different because time is a different experience in hypnosis

Perhaps it begins to seem to you that
you could feel just the same kind of easy,
delightful drifting when you are getting
ready to go to sleep. That would be just
lovely—to feel that secure and very
comfortable sensation. Do you agree?
(*Nods*) You could just *drift* off into sleep,
in the same way that you are enjoying the
sensation of floating in the water right
now. That would be delightful? (*Nods,
sleepily*) Yes. And deep down inside you,
you already know that you will be able to
do that whenever you choose to do so, to
just remember, when you get comfortably
settled in your bed, the same safe
awareness that it is time for you to *drift*
again, to drift off into sleep, and you can
stay in that safe, deep sleep until it is time
to wake up in the morning. Just imagine—
sleeping the whole night through just
as if you were floating in that lovely
warm water, that gently lapped onto the
beautiful little beach—safe, secure sleep,
to awaken in the morning rested and
refreshed.

**Offering the possibility that this
may be adapted in a useful way**

**Suggestions regarding adapting
the floating sensation into sleep**

**Reaffirming that this is possible
and useful, too**

You can use this same experience in your
own hypnosis at home, when you are just
getting ready to go to sleep. You know
how to do it, and you can enjoy that
lovely scene, that delightful sensation,
many, many times, as it carries you into
sleep.

More specific suggestion

Let the client rest for a few more moments.

Now, Jan, you can begin to bring yourself
out of your hypnosis in your own way, as
you know how to do, feeling so refreshed
and calm, knowing that you have learned
something very valuable here today.

**"Knowing that you have
learned" is the key**

*Generally, I find that it is more useful to avoid mentioning anything about the
session, or its possible implications, until the next time your client is in the
office—better to avoid bringing it up into the conscious awareness and just let the
information trickle in, in its own way and its own time.*

Third script: How to spell "sleep"

This is a gimmicky little technique that some people find amusing; others think that it is just nonsense, and therefore not helpful for them. Just let your own perceptions help you to decide whether it would be helpful in any particular case.

Dave, you've mentioned several times that everything about sleeping seems to be difficult for you—falling asleep, staying asleep, and having good quality sleep. This technique that I'm going to describe is a little gimmick that may work for you—perhaps because it *is* just a little gimmick. Are you interested in hearing about it? (*Yes*)

Being up-front that it is, indeed, a gimmick

Alright, then, it goes like this: if you want to help yourself *fall* asleep, make as many words as you can that start from the letters in the word "sleep", that is, s, l, e, e, p. This is different from making new words from rearranging the letters, such as "peels", for example, but all the words you can think of that begin with "s", then "l", then "e" (twice) and then "p". Sometimes people even go around a second time, with words beginning with "sl", then "le", then "ee", then "ep". The possible combinations are almost endless, and often can keep people intrigued until they eventually get tired—or bored—and fall asleep.

Not quite the same as "how many words can you make from the word "Constantinople", but pretty close!

(You may find yourself getting tired—or bored—just describing it!)

Now, to help yourself get *back* to sleep, you do the same thing but with the letters in the phrase, "back to sleep", that is, b, a, c, k, t, o, s, l, e, e, p. You can understand that the opportunities are almost endless.

Getting back to sleep is often more frustrating than getting to sleep in the first place, because you *were* asleep and now you're awake

The third possibility is "all night", or some variation of that thought. You can be your own guide as far as deciding the right way for you to use this rather odd little technique—but then, a lot of things that are really very useful can be thought to be "odd" at times—do you agree? (*Nods*)

One more possibility that needs to be mentioned

Yes. I think so, too. So have fun with this, and you can discover whether you want to use it yourself, as you beckon sleep to come.	**"Have fun" is the essential idea and may seem eminently practical especially while in hypnosis**

Of course, this turns out to be a rather childish game, but remember that when one is in hypnosis, childish games can be a lot of fun, and useful for teaching or introducing a new thought or idea, at the same time. It also takes some of the desperation out of "I have to go to sleep!"

Re-remembering

The following technique is useful for those who are ready to rediscover their own capacity for sleep—falling asleep and staying asleep through the night. It is a play on words and takes some dedication on the part of the therapist! I think that the subconscious mind of the patient often just gets tired of "trying" to decipher what the therapist is saying, and travels off into his or her own dream-like state. It works.

It presumes that the client is either already in hypnosis, or just going into hypnosis, when the script begins.

Mae, we've been talking about using your talent for hypnosis in various ways, to help get past a block, perhaps, or to clarify something.

And there are times when we can use hypnosis to forget something that we have remembered, until it is time to remember to forget. In the same way, we can use hypnosis to remember something that we used to remember and that we now need to remember to remember again—an intriguing kind of *re-remembering*.	**The mind confusion with words begins gently** **The confusion now enters into the texture of the suggestions**

Perhaps it would be interesting to ask that wonderful, subconscious mind of yours to remember how to remember just how wonderful it is to go into sleep— calming, safe, restorative sleep. And perhaps that all-knowing subconscious mind of yours might also be interested in re-remembering something so pleasant and comfortable. Do you think that that might be the case? (*Yes*)

"Remember how to remember …"a strange suggestion

"Re-remembering …" even more strange; but there is no time to consciously decipher the language

Then settle just a little further into your hypnosis, and prepare for an interesting new experience that is actually ages old, remembering to remember.

"ages old …", "remembering to remember …"

And what you can begin remembering to remember, is how delightful it is to fall asleep, to go into that delicious soft, warm, cozy state just before you drift into deep sleep, when you know that that is going to happen and you have the pleasure of the re-remembering of how you did that.

And more of the same …

That's right. Go backwards in time until you reach the time in your life when you first remembered, deep, deep in your *sub-*conscious mind, how to go to sleep. It was so delightful that you were able to forget that you were remembering!

"Backwards in time …"—in other words, remembering

We learn how to do something, and then can forget that we once had to learn it

Take your time, and let me know when, deep in your subconscious mind, you know that you are re-remembering how to remember to go to sleep. (*In a short time, signals*) Yes, that's right. It is truly delightful, that feeling, isn't it? (*Nods*)

Positive suggestion implies that she knows how to do this

Take as long as you wish, in hypnosis
time, to enjoy that awareness, that deep
knowledge that you are re-remembering
what it is like to remember how to go to
sleep. Mmmm. Just drift softly into that **Reinforcing the previous**
lovely, drowsy memory of sleep, also **suggestions, over and over**
knowing that you are re-remembering
how to go to sleep, how to arrive at that
delightful, drowsy, gentle, dreamy time.

You can rest and enjoy, knowing that I will
watch the clock time for you.

*The therapist can softly announce the passing of the clock time—"Now half the
clock time is finished for this part of the hypnosis, now three-quarters of the clock
time is finished…"—until you tell her that the clock time for this part of the
hypnosis is now finished.*

It is time now, in your hypnosis, to **As we can remember how to**
remember how to waken, as you used **remember how to go to sleep,**
to do, gently and comfortably beginning **we can remember how to**
to realize that you are waking up. When **remember how to wake up**
you know, in your hypnosis, that you
are awake, you can bring yourself out of
your hypnosis in your own way, secure **"Secure in the knowledge" is a**
in the knowledge that you have indeed **positive suggestion that things**
re-remembered how to remember how to **have gone well**
go to sleep, and having done that, and re-
remembered, you now know how to go to
sleep when you choose to do so.

Restoring brain chemistry

This may sound rather ominous but it merely consists of plain self-
suggestions that can facilitate the rebalancing of, for example, the serotonin
system (which affects depression) or other biochemical pathways that have
been affected by emotional responses, such as anxiety. As is so often the
case, simple language often works better than sophisticated terminology.

Changes in brain chemistry affect the ability of the client to see past the
present obstacles, for example, or to have sufficient self-assurance that they
can get well. For decades, based on the work with veterans of the Vietnam
War, we believed that these detrimental and intrusive changes in brain
chemistry were permanent. It has taken more than 40 years to discover

that it is not always the case—for some of the veterans, decades later, the chemistry is slowly returning to normal levels. One of the messages that this information offers, is that we need to start paying attention to PTSD biochemical changes as soon as possible, and also that it is never too late to start.

Arthur, we were speaking last week about your depression, which seems to be taking an big emotional toll on you these days. And we also talked about possibly using hypnotic mind–body communication, to help in regulating the biochemical factors in the brain. Are you still interested in exploring that? (*Yes*)

Establishing the use of hypnosis and the purpose or goal

Then just make yourself comfortable, as you have done before, in that nice, comfortable chair here in my office, and go into hypnosis in your own way, to whatever levels seems just right for you this time. Signal when you feel that you are at the right level. (*Signals*)

Settling in

Good. Now you can begin to talk to your own brain—especially that very wise *sub*conscious part of it that is so connected to both mind and body. We've talked before about mind–body communication, and how simple and yet complex that basic communication is. Because of that simple complexity, you can have wonderful inner conversations between all parts of yourself—mind, body, conscious and subconscious—and the physical, emotional, hormonal and biochemical components, too.

Establishing the boundaries in these conversations

"Simple complexity"—hypnospeak
All **the components are essential for positive outcomes**

In fact, these inner conversations can be thought of as exploring all the possibilities, to find the very best pathways towards the rebalancing of all those infinitely precious connections and interactions.

Further justification of the approach

Yet the language itself can be so simple
and straightforward, without all the
jargon that is often used in these
situations.

So just listen to those inner conversations
and translate them, if you wish, into more
simple language that is so much easier to   **Simple is better—and gives the**
understand. For instance, you could say   **client something important to do**
something as simple as "All the important
parts of the equation are coming together
nicely" or "My body understands how to
balance itself, and so does my mind, and
they both know how to do it together."

You can make up a little mantra in your   **You are giving a post-hypnotic**
own words, if you wish, something like   **suggestion**
"All Parts Working Together" or "APWT".
The possibilities are endless but, as you
know, simple often works best.

I'm just going to be quiet now, for a few
moments, and let you do this in your
own, private and personal, way.

*I usually allow about sixty seconds for this; too long, and the patient gets fidgety,
so you have lost an advantage.*

That is very good, Arthur. Do you feel that
this is a good time to come out of your
hypnosis now, and to allow your own
wise subconscious to continue in its own
way? (*Yes*)

Alright. Then just bring yourself back
into this room, comfortably and gently,
knowing that you have done something   **More positive affirmation and**
that was, and is, very important, in your **post-hypnotic strengthening**
work here today.

Rebalancing

Laura, we've been talking about the body's biochemistry getting out of balance when a person has endured terrible trauma, and that something of the sort has probably happened to you. And we were also talking about the body sometimes having a better chance to restore its natural chemistry when hypnosis is used to help that restorative process along. Would you be interested in pursuing that possibility now? (*Yes*)

Establishing the criteria for beginning this process

Alright, this seems like a good time. If, for any reason, you decide that you wish to stop, or put things on hold for a while, you only have to let me know and we can do that. Do you feel comfortable with that?

Knowledge that there is an escape route is always comforting

Good. Then settle yourself into hypnosis, as you know how to do, and let me know when you sense that you are at the right level to begin this work today. (*After a few moments, signals*)

Good. You know that you are ready. Then take yourself backwards in time, back to the time long before the trauma happened, when you were in a good space emotionally and physically, and all seemed right in the world. Again, signal to me when you have that sense. (*Signals*)

Important to establish that she goes backwards in time to well *before* the trauma even began

That's very good. Spend a little time there, in that time, just enjoying the sense of physical and emotional stability. Let your inner self recognize all the factors that contribute to that deep sense of well-being—far more than the cognitive awareness can offer you; somehow, you just *know*.

Allowing time for the awareness to take firm hold

The knowledge is instinctive, not necessarily logical or cognitive

(*After a few moments*) Yes, that's right. You just *know*. Now, knowing that you know, you can come forward in time again into the present time (*mention the present date*), bringing all that knowledge with you. You can just let that happen—your subconscious will help you to do that, so you can allow it to happen in its own way.

Beginning to bring those positive factors into the present

Important that the client *allows* this to happen spontaneously

When you are back in the present (date), ask that wise subconscious mind of yours to begin to reinstate those normal physical and emotional factors so that you are, once again, in a state of total health—in mind, body and spirit—and all functionally well, comfortable and ready to go on with the rest of your life happily and healthily, as you deserve.

The process now continues in its own time, bringing health and well-being—*as you deserve*

"Deserve" is important, because the sense of guilt, in many forms, could otherwise intrude

You may find it interesting, over the next few days and week, to recognize some small—or maybe not so small—changes, all of them letting you know about the good things that are happening. You can smile, then, within yourself, because you will know that your own mind and body are healing. And that's a wonderful knowledge to have.

Reinforcing and reassuring

Rarely is this technique a one-time cure; of course, it is not a cure at all, but rather an opening of the door towards better emotional (biochemical, physiological) health. I usually do a repeat session, using any changes or shifts that the client has told me in our psychotherapy sessions, every couple of weeks until positive progress is established.

Note: The above script may also be used for restoring normal neurophysiology. It is not specifically for that, but could be adapted.

Simple biochemical rebalancing

This script is very simple indeed, and works well when the client doesn't like the idea of "scripts" for getting well.

Dora, I'm going to describe a very, very simple approach to help re-establish normal brain chemistry. You can take yourself into hypnosis if you wish, or just close your eyes and listen.

Whether she is in a "formal" hypnosis or not, her brain will respond as is she were in an altered state of consciousness

When there are times when you would like to speed up the healing process, you might enjoy exploring this short and easy process: just say to yourself, with determination and in a strong and positive voice, "Dora, do what needs to be done to get that biochemistry back in balance!"

The "strong, positive voice" is essential

Say this, in that strong voice, several times a day. You may want to make up a little slogan, or an abbreviation, such as "BIB", meaning "Back in Balance". Some people write short post-it notes to themselves, and put them on the bathroom mirror, or on their desks, or even on the kitchen table—anywhere where the note would catch the eye.

These abbreviations are often very successful, and can be used any time, silently or aloud

Be sure to say it, or read it aloud, at least three times as you get ready to go to sleep. After all, the subconscious can do a lot of its work while we are sleeping.

Saying it just before sleep, is a like a post-hypnotic suggestion

You see? Very simple, as I told you.

Restoring normal neurophysiology

Although the next two scripts may sound as if they would be difficult for the client to fully comprehend, I have found that my clients are perfectly capable of interpreting the message and appreciate the fact that I don't underestimate their intelligence.

Patti, we've talked quite a bit about the brain and about neurophysiology—the science of how the nervous system works—and how mind and body are always in an interaction of some sort with each other. We can be amazed at how complex, and yet how simple that interaction really is.

Setting the scene; you will have discussed this before, at a cognitive level

And we've also talked about the fact that when someone, such as yourself, has endured significant trauma in their life, both the brain chemistry and the neurophysiology are influenced in a major way. The results make up a huge part of what PTSD is all about, as we've also discussed before.

A gentle reminder that she has been through a very difficult time

One thing we also know: that cognitive, rational explanations of PTSD often seem to lack something, although, of course, they help. So it could be that hypnosis might play a bigger role that we used to think in helping the neurophysiology to get back to normal.

Establishing the rationale of using hypnosis

So it often seems like a good idea to explore using some hypnosis. Are you still interested in doing that? (*Yes*)

Good. Then let's start with something simple today, and we can then decide if we want to go into more complex ideas when you've had a chance to ponder on it for a while, between sessions. Does that make sense to you? (*Yes*)

Reassurance that this is going to be something she does know how to do

Then settle in, and comfortably take yourself to whatever level of hypnosis you feel is just right for you, *this* time. (*Signals*)

Now, easily and in your own time, make a sort of map or guide for yourself, that depicts how mind and body are probably interacting at this time in your life, and keeping neurophysiology in mind. This is your own, private map, and nobody needs to see it but you, so you can use whatever symbols or comments you wish.

This is the metaphor I use; knowing your client, you may have a better idea for them

And then, when you have had a chance to do that, and to look at it carefully, make a new map *or* superimpose on the old map whatever new, or different, directions it would be important for you to follow, in order to reach your destination.

This is very important—the opportunity to create a new path towards health

Take your time, and let me know when you have done that to your satisfaction at this time, knowing that it can always be changed later if it seems like a good idea to do that.

Loopholes can be very useful!

Give her time to complete this task, which could take just a few seconds, or may take a few minutes. If more than three or four minutes pass, softly interrupt with a comment such as "That's right—you can be comfortable with that…" and bring her attention back into the room.

That's very good work, Patti. You now have a guide to follow as you allow your subconscious mind to continue the work you have begun here today.

Reassuring her that she has done a good job

And bring yourself out of hypnosis and back into this room, slowly and easily, as you know how to do. You've started something very important, today.

More restoration—another script

This script presumes that you have done something similar to the previous script with your client. However, nothing is written in stone in these pages—they are just guidelines or suggestions to get your own innovative thoughts flowing. So you could, for example, suggest painting a scene, or making up a song, or soaring over the rainbow—or just accessing the richness of your client's imagination. Those riches may seem to be buried, but they're there, or she wouldn't have come this far.

Patti, you did such a good job (last week) when you were here—have you had an opportunity to think about it? (*Yes*)

Making sure that she is still on the same wavelength

There was a suggestion that you might find your own individual way towards restoring *your* personal chart or route to take you to the destination of health in mind and body. And it is so important to help your brain and body find their mutually supportive and healing path. So let's continue with that in mind, shall we? (*Yes*)

We are all different, and have to find that path for ourselves

Mutually supportive is the key phrase here

You can choose whether you want to go into a formal hypnosis, or just relax, close your eyes and allow whatever level of conscious thought seems right, to be there.

She will find her own appropriate altered state of consciousness, in which to do this

(The following presumes that the map, or whatever she used before, is still going to be used.)

So now take another look at that interesting scenario you discovered—created, really—last time. Really look carefully, and find the little sign that says "This is where you can begin to make healthy changes" or "This is where the path can turn in a more positive way". You will know the right way to interpret what I am saying. Let me know when you find that little opportunity, when you have recognized what you need to recognize. (*After a few moments, signals*)

This is a positive hypnotic suggestion to take her to the next level of awareness

"You will know the right way to interpret ..." contains a complex, almost subliminal component

That's very good. Do you realize how well your mind and body are now beginning to collaborate in a very positive way? It's rather amazing—do you agree? (*Yes*)

Affirming that she is doing it right

Everybody has his or her most comfortable way of doing this sort of thing—of the reprocessing and reorganizing patterns of thought and responses that were disrupted because of unexpected, intrusive trauma. It is that reprocessing, that reorganizing, which restores that healthy neurophysiology. You know how to do that, deep down in your wonderful creative, *re*-creative subconscious mind. Begin to trust yourself again, to believe that you do have all the knowledge and skills that you need.

Lots of "re" words that busy the cognitive mind and allow the perceptive right brain to do its innovative work

Because you *do* have them—they have just been temporarily buried underneath the trauma. Let you mind and body do what they know how to do, together, and look towards the secure, positive future that awaits you.

And reaffirming again

Acute Traumatic Stress Disorder

Although we hear more about Post-Traumatic Stress Disorder (PTSD), what happens immediately and up to two or three months after a major traumatic situation creates an equally imperative need for response, and for some tools to combat the fear and anxiety. Such acute event provokes a strong response of fear, helplessness and/or terror.

As with PTSD, there are several recognizable patterns to Acute Traumatic Stress Disorder (ATSD). They are:

- Denial
- Fear
- Concern for personal and family safety
- A subjective sense of numbing or detachment (the physiological equivalent of denial)
- Being in a daze, including derealization and/or depersonalization
- Dissociative amnesia (in some cases)

Dreams, illusions or flashbacks may be prominent, and so the person may do their best to avoid being with others. There may be a tendency to re-live the experience—perhaps to confirm that it was real. In other words, it is an ongoing misery that can last for weeks.

In 2005, scientists in Israel were able to show that blood tests, when taken within hours after the traumatic event, can indicate whether or not PTSD is like to be the eventual outcome. This gives health practitioners an opportunity to stop PTSD before it starts, by understanding ATSD and working for the prevention of further and even more devastating consequences.

Just as the list of the several criteria for PTSD begins with denial, so does the list for ATSD. In fact, at this stage these conditions overlap almost completely. Hypnosis can be helpful in combating the inner turmoil. However, being able to talk about the experience has proven to be invaluable in restoring a sense of reality—that it *did* happen, and that the traumatic response *can* heal.

If the person is able to begin talking about the experience, then reassure them that they can begin to do so, in their own time and in their own way, now. If that is too frightening, though, then hypnosis may pave the way.

First session

Janet, you have had a very disturbing time, and are wondering if the experience really happened, because it seems so surreal. Is that what it's like for you, right now? (*Yes, spoken or indicated*)	**Validating her experience— that it was *real*, not in her imagination**
Yes. Many others, in a similar situation have felt the same way—very disturbed and wondering if it was all a nightmare, and that they'll wake up eventually. (*Nods*)	**Others would feel the same way—more validation**
But you know, in your *logical* mind, that it really did happen, and you are feeling particularly vulnerable. That's normal, for such a disturbing experience. Do you agree? (*Nods*)	**Normalizing her response to the situation**
So let us think on that for a little while. We could, for example, ask your logical mind and your perceptual mind to have a communication, each asking for the other's response and finding out where or if those responses might coalesce, or distance themselves. Would that be that be alright? (*Nods*) Good.	**Suggesting a means of regaining a sense of control. This is very important, because with acute trauma, one feels *out of* control**

Then I'm going to suggest a way to do
this, but if you think of a better way, then
it is your choice, because, of course, this
is *your* hypnosis, rather than mine, and it
needs to be just right for you. (*Nods*)

Let your subconscious mind and your
conscious mind have a communication.
That might be through words, sensation,
emotion, or whatever those very intricate   **Down to practicalities: how can**
and special parts of your brain feel is just   **one achieve this?**
the right way to achieve that connection.
Ask that wonderful mind of yours to
somehow give you a signal that this is
happening. Let me know when you have   **The presumption is: you *can* do**
such a perception. Take your time. I'll   **it!**
watch the clock time for you.

(*She indicates that this has happened.*)

That is very good indeed. Remember to   **This is a deliberate distraction,**
say "thank you" to your wonderful mind,   **to prevent her from going too**
for helping you in this way.   **far into the *process* of what is**
                                                  happening, but simply just
                                                  accepting it

Now, just allow that communication to
grow, and let it send you a message, in
some way, to indicate that that is what is
happening. Signal to me when you know
that you have received that message.

(*Allow time for this to happen. If it seems to be taking a long time, make a
confirmatory sound, such as "Um-hum, that's right."*)

Yes, I think that you are beginning to recognize some shift, some change that is positive for you, and somehow bring a little relief. It may be just a relaxing of your muscles, or breathing seems a bit easier. You can recognize the signals. In fact, you could take a deep breath and find out how it feels. That's right, good. Continue to let your muscle tightness ease, and feel yourself regaining as sense of control. It's funny, how letting tightness go can help you feel stronger. Perhaps you feel that, too.

Straightforward suggestion that a shift is happening. Look for any signal that she is rejecting this—but she will more likely accept the implied demand. You are suggesting a paradox, by simultaneously easing muscle tightness and feeling stronger, more in control

Janet, I think that you are already feeling better. Do you feel that too? (*Nods*) Excellent. You have been doing some very good work, today. Are you ready to come out of your hypnosis now? (*Nods or says "Yes"*)

Good. Then just bring yourself back, in your own way, and when you are ready, open your eyes.

Be sure to congratulate her on a job well done. She may feel a little spacey, but your reassurance will be very important. Usually it is a good idea to arrange another appointment quite soon, within a few days at the most. She may request a therapy session—you can discuss this with her but wait for her to make the suggestion. Perhaps she might feel, tentatively, that she is ready to start talking about it. If so, let her begin, and support her while she struggles to find words to describe it. If she is not ready to put it all into words yet, just offer reassurance that she has already begun the healing process and will be able to talk about it soon. This can be reinforced in the next hypnosis session.

Second session

You have been doing a little catch-up, letting her tell you what it has been like for the past few days, If she says that she is still quite distracted or panicky, a simple reinforcing "you can do it" session might be in order. You can remind her that she is safe, there in your office. Just do a simple relaxation session, with positive suggestions about being proud of herself.

If, however, she is ready to strengthen the last session and proceed, you can go forward.

Janet, you have been telling me that you have been managing more comfortably during the few days since our last session. Is that right? (*Yes*)

Reaffirming progress

Good for you. Do you still sense that communication that you recognized last time, between your conscious, logical mind and your subconscious, perceptual mind? (*Nods*) That's excellent. You can feel very proud of yourself.

Reinforcing her own capability

Do you feel ready to go further, now? (*Nods*) Very good. You are making excellent progress.

A suggestion buried in a question

So let yourself recognize where you want to go from here. To a further, stronger communication between your conscious and your subconscious mind? Or perhaps on to an entirely new stage of healing. I'll offer those two possibilities one at a time, and you can signal, or tell me, which you prefer.

Clarifying the two suggestions can make the decision process easier

FIRST CHOICE: A STRONGER COMMUNICATION

Then you can say, to that strong mind of yours, that enhancing the communication between the conscious and the sub-conscious can offer new perspectives for the healing process, and suggest that these various new perspectives can now begin to become apparent to both the conscious and subconscious parts of your brain.

Repeating "strong" is reassuring and relaxes any hypervigilance, paving the way for possible new perspectives

"Conscious and subconscious" is also reassuring

SECOND CHOICE: READY TO GO ON TO A NEW STAGE OF HEALING

Then thank that strong mind of yours for the work that it has been doing, and tell both your conscious and your subconscious that you are ready to go to the next stage of healing.

Always useful to offer thanks to oneself

Be specific in your acknowledgement of all that good work, and nod when you know that your appreciation has been received. (*After a little time, nods*) Yes, that's right.

Reaffirming

The next stage of healing can be a clearer recognition of the event(s), and a clear knowledge that you were innocent for what happened. It is important to be *very* clear about that, because then you can put those events into that realistic perspective, which is so important.

Entering the next stage

Making everything very clear!

Repetition in hypnosis is strengthening

Now you are ready to process all those event(s), step by step, stage by stage. You can take as much time as you need for this, and so it is often useful to bring yourself out of hypnosis being confident that your wise brain will continue to work on this important step.

Post-hypnotic suggestion that the healing process has begun and will continue

Continuing and regular sessions will almost certainly be needed for the next few weeks. They can be short hypnosis sessions, as part of a regular psychotherapy session, or longer ones dedicated to the hypnosis, separate from the therapy sessions.

Any time she indicates that she is ready to put it all into words, or to tell you more that she has remembered, give her time to do that.

Further processing

Janet, you have been making excellent progress. I'm thinking that there may be some particular situation that you would like to understand better—maybe the way you responded, or the way it actually evolved. Am I right in that assumption? (*Signals "Yes"*)

Setting the scene for further work

Then settle now, into whatever level of
hypnosis you mind will instinctively
recognize as just the right level for this to
happen, and let me know when you are at
that place. (*After a few moments, nods*) Very
good.

And now, let your awareness go to that
particular situation. You might see it, hear
it, sense it—some perceptual response that
lets you know you are at that time and
place. Let me know when you experience
that. (*After a time, nods*) That's right, very
good.

**Remember that much of this is
perceptual rather than cognitive
language-and-logic recognition,
and therefore that this is an
indication (rather than a logical
decision) that she is ready to
make that shift**

When you are able, begin to tell me
what is now happening, what you are
experiencing.

*As she begins to do that, allow her lots of time to express what she is perceiving.
It is often difficult to put it into words, but to put it into words is exactly what
she needs to do. In the meantime, you simply offer "helpful noises", as one of
my colleagues, Dr Clair Frederick, used to say: "um-hum", "ohhh", a-ha". It is
alright to softly ask that she explain a bit more, but she may or may not be able do
that. Phrases such as "I see ..." and "That seems important—is it?" can be useful,
too. But it is crucial that she put it into words, not you.*

When you sense that it is a good time to stop for now, you can say:

You have been doing wonderfully well,
Janet. Perhaps this would be a good
time to let it rest for now, so that that
wonderful brain of yours can get it all into
the new context. Would that be alright?
(*Nods*)

**Positive reinforcement is very
important, but so is letting her
have time to process the new
perception(s)**

Good. Then in your own time, come out
of your hypnosis, bringing with you that
positive awareness that you have begin
a whole new part of the healing process,
today.

*Usually it is important to give the client time to fully process these changes.
Remember that there has been significant trauma and, although some recover more
quickly than others, it is important that we allow that time. The client will let you
know if and when they feel ready to move on.*

Self-worth

Even those people with a strong sense of self-worth—that innate belief that "I am worthy simply because I *am*: I exist, I am a person, a human being, doing my best"—find that it is difficult to be so sure about their worthiness when they have been in a traumatic situation.

Self-worth is different to self-esteem, which has to do with achievements. Self-esteem is very important, too, but it has different roots than the sense of self-worth. Self-worth begins at a very early age—even, we now think, before birth: maternal hormones may somehow begin the process of believing oneself worthy. The pregnant woman who is joyous that she is going to have a child *may* be offering that child more than she realizes.

After birth, the simple actions of a parent (usually the mother, but not always or necessarily) in reassuring and strengthening that sense by hugs and cooing and smiling and tone of voice, offers that young human being the awareness of worthiness. It is, at this stage, implicit; it will be several years before the explicit becomes important. By the time that is happening, self-esteem possibilities are presenting themselves, too. Perhaps one of the best examples of the difference is the highly acclaimed movie star who decides that her life isn't worth living and commits suicide. She may have acquired considerable self-esteem, and well-earned, too, but has virtually no sense of self-worth.

Strong self-esteem does not offer the same protection from trauma that self-worth offers. Nevertheless, trauma can, and often does, erode that sense of self-worth because the victims frequently blame themselves for the event—"If only I had been more careful …", "If only I had seen it coming …", "If only I hadn't been so stupid …" etc.

Bill, we've talked in the past about how trauma affects our sense of self. Very often people feel that they are to blame for what happened, and this erodes that deep and positive knowledge, so very essential to one's personal worthiness. Perhaps you have been feeling that way yourself (*Nods, or says "Yes" or signals*)	**Normalizing the situation**
Then let's focus on that important aspect. Are you comfortable with doing that today? (*Nods*) Good.	**It is important that he is ready to start this part of the process**

Go deep within yourself, then, to that core of self. You will know when you have reached that destination. Take your time—sometimes it takes a person a little longer; others reach that place more quickly. I'll just stay quiet, and you can let me know when you have reached that sense of self. (*In time, he signals or says, "Yes"*)

Ideomotor responses, e.g. finger-lifting, are also helpful and require less conscious decision-making

That's very good.

Now, look at yourself clearly, because you can do that, and find out what you need to know about your sense of self-worth at this difficult time in your life. Some people find it helpful to envision a scale, or some sort of yardstick, that helps them to gain that perspective.

The positive, declarative way of speaking is reassuring

For example, you might think of your sense of self-worth—your own very *personal* sense of self-worth—on a scale of 1 to 10, and allow your subconscious to place the pointer on the right number. Let me know when you have found that number.

Making sure that it is personal, and that it is the *subconscious* that sets that number

(*Signals. This may take several moments—that is normal*)

Now, gradually improve that number on the scale, as much as you feel ready to improve it right now. Let me know when you have done that. And you can improve it as little, or as much, as just feels right for you at this time.

Often, he is only ready to go up one number, or even half a number. Whatever it is, congratulate the client

Now, you may feel that you would just like to stay at that level for a while—maybe even a day or so, until you are ready to look at it again and perhaps improve it another notch. But this is *your* sense of self-worth, and it is *your* time of changing or not changing it, that is important.

Saying this will actually improve the sense of self-worth, because it is the client who is making the decision, not the therapist

You have been doing good work. Are you now ready to come out of your hypnosis? (*Yes*) Then bring yourself out of hypnosis, back into this room, in your own way.	**This establishes his own capability to make the decision, and follow through**

In subsequent sessions, inquire about self-worth in a calm way, as if you are simply asking about the weather. If you sense some erosion, then reinforce the message in this script by repeating it in hypnosis.

Physiological response to trauma

This subject was discussed in an earlier section of the book.

Basically, to review: after trauma headaches, poor sleep or insomnia, aches and pains of unknown origin (and unlikely to be caused by a physical problem), sweats, nightmares and similar disturbances of day-to-day functioning are very common.

It doesn't matter whether, to someone else, the trauma seems sufficient to cause such a problem—the fact is that the symptoms are there. Women may find that their menstrual cycle is upset; both men and women may find that their sexual function and response are affected. Tempers may surge for no apparent reason, and relationships consequently may suffer. I mentioned in the earlier section on ATSD (page 77), that numbing, a sense of detachment or an apparent absence of emotional responsiveness, are common.

All of these need to be discussed openly with both the family physician and the therapist. Once the person has been cleared of physical clinical problems, then hypnosis can help. (Of course, hypnosis can also be helpful if there *are* physical clinical problems, but that is a different situation.)

We can use *numbing* as an example of this kind of mind–body communication—a communication that appears to produce a negative result, but which can be useful as an introduction into the role that hypnosis can play—a helpful entrance towards healing. Remember that numbing can be emotional, physical or both.

First script

Ellen, you've told me that you are bothered by this sense of emotional numbness that is staying with you. Would you like to use hypnosis to ease that? (*Yes*)

Establishing the situation

Alright. Then just make yourself as comfortable as you can at this time, and go into hypnosis in your own way, to whatever level feels just right for you today. Let me know when you have reached that level. (*Signals*)

That's very good. Just spend a little time by clock time—as long as you like in hypnosis time—as you become more and more comfortable in thought and in your body.

Giving her time to settle

Um-hum. Now, focus for a moment on the numbness, just for a moment, so that you can recognize all its qualities.

Avoid too much attention on the problem, but important to recognize the experience

That's right. Now is the time—when you have just recognized these qualities—to ask your subconscious mind and your body to work together, and to collaborate, in a way that brings more ease.

This is an essential step—the mind–body collaboration

And as your mind and body begin to do that, be aware of those tiny shifts of sensation that indicate a change. They may be *very* small shifts, so be sure to pay attention and go slowly, but very intently, as this shifting begins to happen.

Easing into the possibility of relief; at times, relief is frightening—something new and strange is happening

You might notice a sight awareness of some particular part of your body, a hand, perhaps, or your face. It may even seem as if that part of your body is coming to visit you again, after having been away for a while.

Down-to-earth examples are comforting

She may nod or give some indication that something like that is happening.

Yes, I think you sense that something like that is just beginning to happen. Your mind and your body are now communicating, just as you asked them to do.	**Reassurance that all is evolving as it should**
Now that you know that that wonderful subconscious mind of yours, and your body, can focus together on those new, strange experiences, and together can begin to heal, you have taken a new step. You can, in your own hypnosis and your own time, continue to ask for this communication between your mind and your body, because now you know that it can really happen.	**Positive reinforcement**

Of course, this script is just an example, but it can be a basis for exploring the mind–body interaction, and that this is a positive thing to recognize.

Second script

Jason, you've told me that you are quite concerned because you "don't seem to feel any more". I'm presuming that you mean that you have no emotional response, or very little. Is that right?	**Clarifying the situation**
And I think that you are wondering if this means that there is something wrong with you. Am I also right in that assumption?	**Further clarification**
It's important, therefore, to find some way to reassure yourself that this is another part of what "getting over trauma" means. You may even prefer to think of it as getting around it, or pushing through it. So will it be alright to explore a bit, through hypnosis? (*Yes*)	**Important to reassure that people "get over trauma" in different ways and with different timing**
Good. Settle in a little deeper, then, to whatever level feels comfortable at this time. Let me know when you have reached that level. (*Nods*)	

So you have a very keen understanding of how the "right level" feels. That is an excellent start.

A new perspective!

Now that you are somewhat reassured that you are doing it right, take a few deep breaths and allow yourself to go a little further into hypnosis if you wish. Um-hum. That's right.

Giving an opportunity to take the next step

Now go even further back in your clear memory bank, to a long time before the trauma even happened, when you had a strong emotional response to some situation. It doesn't matter what the situation was—it only matters that you recognize the strong emotional response. Let me know when that happens. (*After a little time, nods*)

Finding a link

Excellent. Now you know for sure that you are indeed capable of experiencing that strong emotional response. It helps to know that. Do you agree? To *really* know that? (*Nods—may give a sigh of relief*)

Reassurance—he is indeed capable of feeling, after all

Yes, it does help to know that.

And now you also know something else: that that wise subconscious mind of yours has been keeping your deep emotional responses safe, while you are coming to terms with what happened.

Offering a rational explanation, that the hypnotic state will decipher in its own way

And now you are ready to know that you can let your subconscious know, that you are getting ready to allow yourself to experience the emotional *response* again—starting slowly, while you become re-accustomed to feeling those emotions as you used to, before the trauma. (*May sigh, or nod*)

Hypnospeak: his subconscious deciphers it as he needs to, and in its own time

Be comfortable with that knowledge. You can be very interested in perceiving how your ability to feel those feelings begins to return.

More hypnospeak: very useful as it allows *him* to decipher what "perceiving" means to him

Now, let yourself come out of your hypnosis in your own way, reassured that you have moved forward, in a positive way, today.

He may be wondering what has happened, but he can be reassured that is was good— whatever it was!

Critical Incident Stress Disorder

My personal definition of this disorder is that some particular incident, often one that occurred in the line of duty (fire-fighters, emergency response teams, police) was the essential factor in creating the situation. Typical situations include assault (often in the line of duty), other forms of abuse, life-threatening potential, serious injury—to oneself or another colleague—and also those situations which have a high publicity potential.

Critical Incident Stress Disorder (CISD) almost always has to do with the person's perception of their own ability to cope with a specific situation, and the level of emotional reaction that it evoked.

Whether or not a situation is likely to result in CISD depends on a range of factors, which include exhaustion, frustration, a feeling of helplessness ("I couldn't stop it …"), and also the length of time involved and the level of personal risk. Mitigating factors can include advance warning, previous experience, and professional support immediately afterwards and on-going.

As is so often the case in trauma situations, the mind alternates between denial and intrusive thoughts. In the best scenarios, this process will eventually allow the person to integrate the trauma in a positive way. If, however, there is no time to do this, then a Critical Incident Stress Disorder is in the making. The ability to *cope* with the situation efficiently is a more important factor in ameliorating the descent into CISD.

Our brains are programmed to imprint events; the brain therefore does its best to place a new input within those imprinted perspectives—for example, is this new event or circumstance associated with previous similar situations or emotional responses, or is it notably different from previous experiences? In one situation it may be more in the realm of cognitive thinking, in another it is more connected to previous emotional perceptions. If something happens—an unexpected stimulus of some sort, a sense, a smell—this usual process is disrupted and the burgeoning memory skitters around unfettered. The core site of memory processing—the hippocampus, which can be thought of as a bridge between perception and logic—can *mis*perceive, and a critical incident is formed.

As with Acute Traumatic Stress Disorder, early opportunity to debrief is very important. Such a debriefing would include facts (logic), thought (perception) and reaction (response, symptoms, including physiological response), and these are all areas where hypnosis can be useful. Remember, though, that the final outcome is determined by the ability to put it into words. Until this is achieved, the possibility of developing Acute Traumatic Stress Disorder and/or Critical Incident Stress Disorder remains high.

As I indicated in the previous paragraphs, a significant element in critical stress response is *misperception*. This leads to the brain being blocked from processing the information properly, and may therefore result in the brain acting as if the incident is continuing. The person therefore continues to respond as if the incident is still happening. In addition, there is another misperception—that the event was somehow normal but that the individual experiencing the stress was/is somehow abnormal. Workers involved in such a situation may begin to assume that somehow the fault lies with them.

You may like to begin with a pre-hypnosis conversation in order to get the story straight:

"Joe, you have told me about the very difficult circumstances around this event, and that you were unable to save the woman who was trapped. Is that right?"

"Yes. I didn't do my job properly. If I had, she may have survived."

"Yet your comrades, and even your Superior Officer, have said that you did everything you could have done."

"Yes, but they were just trying to make me feel better."

"So you don't believe them?"

"No. They're nice guys, but they're just being kind."

"You know, because we've talked about it, that our brains process very stressful situations *perceptually* rather than logically."

"Yes."

"Would it be alright, then, to approach this from a perceptual point of view and then see if your logical perspective might be different? And could we use hypnosis as a framework for that?"

"If you want. But it won't change anything."

"Let's see if hypnosis might help. Even a little relief would be better—do you agree?"

"Yes, but—"

(Note: He may already be in an altered state of consciousness because of his intense connection to the situation. Going into hypnosis is an easy transition.)

Settle back into the chair then, and let your eyes close if that is comfortable for you. That's right.	**Settling him into hypnosis; use whatever approach is applicable**
(Give him time to do this.)	
Now, take yourself back to an hour or so *before* the situation seemed to get out of hand. Things seemed to be going as smoothly as possible under the circumstances. Notice all the usual things that you do in those situations, and that you are doing those very things as you always do. Just slowly go through those usual steps. You're doing them the way you have learned to do them. Is that right? (*Yes*)	**He is doing all the usual things—all the things he has been taught how to do**
So, you know that you are proceeding as you have been taught, as you have learned in the past. Just go through those steps, one by one.	**This is very important**

As frequently happens, he has jumped forward in time and is beginning to get agitated. This happens when the emotional factor seems to get ahead of the logical factor. We need to be prepared for it.

(*Beginning to get agitated*) Joe calls out: "This isn't going right! This isn't going right!"

"Why is it not going right?"

"Because—because she isn't talking—she should be talking to me!"

"And why can't she, Joe?"

"Because …"

At this point, Joe is realizing that there is a reason why the woman isn't responding (or whatever the situation is) and that her lack of response is because of some situation that had already happened before Joe got there. This is the basis for a shift in perspective—that he was not responsible for her lack of response.

Yes, Joe. Go back now, to what you were telling me before things seemed to get out of hand. Tell me about it again.

You are taking him back through the steps again, to reinforce that he *has* been doing it right

You may need to go through several repeats as he comes to terms with the new information his brain is now computing, with logic, to offset the previous perceptual belief. In fact, he had done all the things that he had been taught to do.

Obviously, this is just one scenario; other situations will inevitably be different. But the approach is the same: in hypnosis, help the client to go back to the beginning of the event, preferably before the situation turned bad, when things were going as they should, and they are telling you about what happened, putting it all into words, to facilitate the shift from emotion to logic.

Obsessive-Compulsive Disorder

People who regularly deal with emergency situations, often have specific (some would say unique) personality traits—for example, the ability to shut out everything that is going on around them, or a single-minded dedication to one particular aspect of a situation. So strong is their determination to perform in a certain way, that for some it becomes obsessive, and sometimes, that's a good thing. Generally, these traits serve them well, allowing them to get on with the job at hand without needing to dissect it. This certainly applies to fire-fighters, police, ambulance drivers, military personnel and others who serve in these and similarly demanding occupations.

One of these traits is the need to perform perfectly (obsessive) and another—often linked—is to be able to repeat the same actions over and over again (compulsive). Of course, these can be found in other people and situations too, and can, at times, be linked back to personal trauma and the need to do everything perfectly so that the same desperate situation is avoided. Some adaptation of the following scripts can be utilized in either case.

First session

Mark, you've told me that you are sick and tired of always feeling overwhelmed by your obsessive thoughts, and we have discussed the possibility that hypnosis may help. Are you ready to explore that possibility now? (*Yes*) Good.

Important to make sure that he is ready to help himself

You many wish to choose a certain type of situation in which these thoughts impose on you, and use that as a way to begin changing. Do you have some particular obsession that you would like to focus on? (*Yes*) Alright, that's fine. It often helps to be specific.

Usually it is best to have some specific situation in mind, as a starting point

Then let yourself begin to experience those very obsessive thoughts, but only in a very small way, as if you were at the edges rather than in the middle of such thoughts. Let me know when that is happening. (*Nods or other message e.g. ideomotor signal*)

It is helpful to keep the situation as minor as possible to begin with

Begin to separate out the obsessive thought into its various parts—because there are always various parts—for example, how you first become aware that this obsessive thought is present. A sensation? A trigger word? Maybe something you see or hear? Nod when you find such a part. (*After a pause, he nods*)

This gives him something to do, which is almost always helpful because it directs—or re-directs—his focus

Now that you have found such a part, you can begin to let it change, become smaller, or perhaps paler, so that it sends a weaker message. It's just a *little* part of the response.

Generally, the smaller the change, the more likely it is to take effect

Because we know that when one part of a situation changes, other parts often begin to change too, it is just fine to see whether that happens spontaneously after you have made this little change. Let's see what evolves, in both your subconscious and in your conscious mind. We can talk about this at your next session, your thoughts and your feelings, and discuss how you may choose to proceed from there.

Because obsessions become so ingrained, it is usually more helpful to adopt this bit-by-bit approach

In the meantime, you may find it very interesting to observe any shifts in your thoughts or your responses to events going on around you.

Next session

Mark, you have told me that the obsession seems a little less intrusive—is that right? (*Yes*) And that is very encouraging. You know now that you can make the changes that are important for you. Are you ready to make another small change, or shift, today? (*Yes*)

Accentuate the positive!

Good. Then you can either focus on the same part, and continue to lessen its impact on you, or choose another, whichever feels best for you.

Implicit reassurance that he can make more progress

After several sessions, he will become even more assured that he can, in fact, lessen the impact of the obsession on his life; then you and he can choose to continue with another "small thing", or just let those small shifts evolve in their own way. You and he have already set the stage for further changes.

Another example

Susan, we have often talked about your compulsive behaviour, and how it really interferes with your day-to-day life, and you have indicated that you want to change. Would you like to start that process today? (*Yes*)

Making sure that she is ready

Alright. Choose one of your compulsions, one that is fairly minor to begin with. Can you make a choice? (*Yes*) Good.

Starting with a minor choice is more likely to be useful

Let yourself be aware of that compulsion, and begin to reassure yourself, over and over, that you *can* change. Maybe you can repeat it less often each time, or set some sort of new, softer criteria that allow you to become more in charge of that behaviour. It is always a good thing to feel more in charge, by making the changes that are useful.

This is almost an invitation to open a new compulsion; be careful, and observe your client carefully. Remember, the compulsive behaviour *does* give the perception of being in charge, to accent the "useful changes"

Start with a very small change and tell yourself, over and over, that you can do that, that you can take charge of that little change. Reassure yourself that you *can* do that, and create a useful change.

This is rather like trading one compulsion for an other, but it often works, and the alliteration will help, too (change/charge/change)

Practice this all week, and stay positive. Just go with the repetitive phrases. You can do it!

Arrange to see her again next week; softening compulsions doesn't come easily, so you need to be very reassuring. Whether she has had some apparent success or not, congratulate her for her determination.

Anxiety disorders

We can think in terms of three different types of anxiety disorder:

(1) Reactive anxiety—related to some particular incident; the fear of another such incident can be overwhelming.
(2) Conditioned anxiety—the person continues to be triggered by old fears, to the extent that day-to-day behaviour is impaired. The client may be experiencing forgetfulness, insomnia, or other similar intrusions into everyday life.
(3) Free-floating anxiety—very difficult to cope with because there seems to be no reason for the anxiety. There is therefore nothing to hang it on and apparently no starting point for reducing the impact.

Anxiety disorders disrupt the daily activities of life, often in a very intrusive way. They cause sleep disturbances, inability to perform as expected, (e.g. in the workplace), loss of the ability to temper anger and also loss of the ability to understand the source of the anger, difficulty concentrating because they are concentrating on the anxiety instead, and a greatly diminished sense of self-worth.

Reactive anxiety

One would think that this would be the easiest to treat, but that is not always the case. We need to realize that this type of anxiety, so limited in its boundaries, can be a major cause of disruption in the person's life. It can certainly become obsessive. Some sufferers become quite hypervigilant in an effort to never encounter the same circumstances again.

Alice we have been talking about the phobia you have about birds. You have told me how it all began, many years ago, when you were frightened as a child. We talked about using hypnosis to help you cope, because this problem does interfere in your life a great deal. You like to go for walks, but are afraid to because you might have another bad experience with birds. And it is even hard for you to visit friends who keep pet birds, even though the birds are in cages. Does that describe your situation? (*Yes*)	**Setting the scene** **The reason for using hypnosis** **Wanting a return to normalcy**

Are you ready then, to see if hypnosis can help? (*Yes*)

Be sure that she is still in agreement

Good. So settle into that comfortable chair, and let yourself begin to release a little of that tension in your muscles. Some people like to release it all at once, through breathing or in some other way, and some choose to go through their bodies systematically, easing the tension as they go from head to toe. You can release that tension in your own way, so just begin, You can close your eyes, knowing that you are safe, in my office.

Giving her time to settle, and release tension in her body (and therefore also in her mind)

(*She begins to let some of the tension go.*) That's right; good—you are doing that very well.

Now go deep inside yourself, and find that little girl who was so frightened when the bird came at her. She didn't know what to do, did she? And there was nobody there at that moment to help her. You can ease her distress now. Let her tell you all about it; you can reassure her that you really understand why she was so frightened. I'll be quiet for a little time, so that she can tell you. You can let me know when she has done that. (*After a few minutes, she nods*)

Accessing the "little girl" (we all have our "young parts" within us and it is a useful metaphor)

She is putting the adult in charge of the situation

Yes. She was very frightened. You were able to help her, I think. (*Nods*) That's very good.

Reaffirming that the adult helped the child

So now you know that you have been able to comfort her; you can let her know that she can always come to you if she needs to be comforted or reassured. You can do that; is that right? (*Nods*) Yes, I thought so. So now you now you also know that when you feel frightened about birds, that is just the little girl telling you that she is frightened, and you can comfort her and reassure her that you're there, and you're a grown-up, so then she can feel safe.

You are taking it for granted that she will be able to do that; because she is in hypnosis, the odds are high that she will accept that conclusion. "You're a grown up ..." insinuates that she will take on that role

That is very good work. Perhaps you can speak with her again before we close for today, and reassure her that you will be there for her any time she needs to be comforted.

This sets the scene for future work, if it is needed

This general pattern is infinitely variable to fit into almost any situation where the sense of personal competence needs bolstering. The adult can always be there to help the child. It fosters the belief that, "I am the adult now, and I can help the child part of me that is having trouble with this ..." and it certainly strengthens the sense of self-worth.

Conditioned anxiety

This type of anxiety is, of course, very similar to reactive anxiety, but on a much broader base. While taking the history, you will acquire a good idea of the scope of this anxiety disorder. The actual details do not matter as much as the fact that there are many triggers for the anxiety response.

It is important to find out as much as you can about the various triggers and the bank of responses the client uses. Many clients suffer psychosomatic responses and are insulted with the presumption that "It's all in your head". Of course, it is, but (as I have said before) that doesn't mitigate the distress; in fact, it adds to it, and the client is somehow made to feel incompetent.

One of my basic ploys is to use the same technique as I described for reactive anxiety—i.e. the adult comes to help the child. Just adapt the script to suit the broader response.

Another technique is to use the "Mind–Body Communication, Collaboration, Cooperation" scenario and adapt it to the client's specific needs. I had one female client who went around muttering "MBCCC, MBCCC, MBCCC" over and over again until the worst of the anxiety response was subdued. The important element was that she knew that she could control it that way.

Another technique is to go systematically through the body, releasing tension as you encounter it.

Kate, I know that you want to reinforce some of the hypnotic techniques that are so useful when anxiety strikes. Is that right? (*Yes*)

Setting the program

Then take yourself into hypnosis in your own way, and we can get started. Let me know when you feel that you are at the right level for you today. (*After a short pause, she signals*) Very good.

Now begin by focusing on your head, releasing the muscle tension in your scalp. You know how to do that. Nod when you have released that tension. (*Nods*) Good. Now, across the forehead and around the temples. Around the eyes, of course. Around the nose and ears—important to remember that—around the mouth, and over and under the chin and jaw. Very good.

This whole script is an invitation to deliberately release muscle tension in the whole body, from head to toe

Now down the back of the scalp and the back of the neck That's right. Around the shoulders, and down the arms. Though the elbows, down the arms then through the hands and right out through the fingertips. Excellent.

Now down through the trunk of the body, back and front, inside and out. Remember how much muscle there is *inside* the body! The heart, of course, is a muscle; there are tiny muscle fibers in the respiratory tree; the walls of the intestine are muscle. These are different kinds of muscle, of course, but those muscles deserve to be comfortable, too. So through the diaphragm—another muscle—and down to the muscles of the lower back. These are very important muscles. They hold us up.

Continuing the encouragement

Through the abdomen and pelvis and
down the thighs—back and front,
remember—these muscles are very
important, as they also hold us up.
Through the knees, down the legs,
through the ankles and the feet and out
through the toes.

And you have released muscle tension
right through your whole body! We call it
"progressive relaxation".

You did that very well indeed. Just spend
another few moments enjoying the new
sensations in your body of comfortable
relaxation, yet still very aware of the
muscles and the excellent work that they
do. And now say "thank you" to yourself
for doing that exercise.

**You may want to emphasize
"new sensations"**

You may also realize that when we release
muscle tension, we release emotional
tension, too! Just check and see whether
that is true for you, now.

**Usually the client will smile and
say, "Oh, yes—I can feel that,
too!"**

So now you know how to do that—to
release tension right through your body
and also in your emotional self at the
same time. You can practice this very
simple technique. And you could also
give yourself a code word that would
immediately invite your mind and
body to enjoy the this tension-releasing
experience. Just give yourself that code
word, now. Keep it private—it is your
own *special* code word.

**You are giving her a post-
hypnotic suggestion, although
she may not realize it**

Now, in your own time, bring yourself out
of your hypnosis, and enjoy feeling that
relief.

**Another post-hypnotic
suggestion**

Note: Many people are more receptive to post-hypnotic suggestions when
they are just on the verge of coming out of hypnosis. It is as if the "logic
guard" at the gate has left his post for a little while.

Along the same lines, but more directed to the specific symptoms (rapid heart beat, short gasping breaths, clutching sensations in the gut, etc.) more suggestions can be found in the emotional pain section on page 13. It is very easy to adapt it to the needs of someone suffering severe panic and anxiety.

Free-floating anxiety

This is probably the most difficult type of anxiety to treat because it *is* "free-floating" and therefore almost impossible to pin down. There seems to be no obvious reason for the anxiety— it is not related to any event or set of circumstances—and because of this it is difficult to treat. Anxiety becomes a constant interference in the person's life for no apparent reason; the symptoms can arise seemingly out of nowhere. Often, the "no apparent cause" is, in itself, cause for further panic and anxiety. The client may be reluctant to go out—especially to social events—for fear that they will suddenly become completely incapacitated, unable to speak clearly or cogently, unable to describe what's really wrong but feeling an imperative need to get away.

When asked about any past trauma in their lives, clients with this disorder will be unable to pinpoint any situation that could be the root of the anxiety. Nevertheless, there must have been a cause at some previous time in their lives for this problem to have become so interfering in what would ordinarily be called "normal" activities. Even the most innocuous of experiences can become malignant and disproportionately intrusive. An in-depth history is very important.

First session

Laura, you have been suffering from this free-floating kind of anxiety for so long, it must be interfering in your day-to-day life to a considerable degree. (*Yes*)

Stating the obvious—but it sets the scene

You have found that medication seems useless—maybe it even makes things more exasperating—so we must look for another approach. We have talked about hypnosis. Do you feel that you would like to explore that now? (*Yes*)

Rationale for using hypnosis

Then settle into hypnosis in your own way, as you know how to do. You also know that you are safe, here in my office, so you can be comfortable, and can enjoy yourself in your own very special place.

Establishing the safety of the present situation

(*When she has settled down*) Now, allow yourself to feel just the tiniest bit of that pervasive anxiety that you so often have— just the *tiniest* bit. That's right. And hold it there, at that tiny bit.

This can be tricky, so be firm about the *tiniest* bit, and backtrack if you suspect that it is too much

Maybe that tiny bit of anxiety is looking for a safe place, too. So you can talk to it, privately, and find out if that might be the case.

A different role for the anxiety! (And one that would only work in hypnosis)

Yes, that's right—let that very tiny bit of anxiety have its role understood, too! Use your wonderful, bright imagination and give that anxiety its own place in the spectrum. *That's* right—go on with that idea.

Using a strange collaboration of logic and metaphor—it often works

Now listen carefully to what that little anxiety part is telling you. Perhaps it might even have an idea of its own as to how you can both feel better. Let me know when this is happening. (*Give her time to work this through*)

Hypnotic suggestion can ignore reality; you are suggesting a major shift in perception to get across a cognitive barrier

That's very good indeed, Laura. It is wonderful how the subconscious can help—do you agree? You can take that new knowledge home, where it can have further subconscious processing. Let's make an appointment for next week, so we can reassess the situation. Will that be alright? (*Yes*) Good. You have done some excellent work today.

Reinforcing the positive

Laura will probably need several more sessions, similar to this, until she feels—at last—that she is in control rather than the anxiety being in control. The next script will offer some suggestions about that.

Second session

Laura, you had an interesting experience last time you were here, when a tiny part of the anxiety response seemed to take on a different perspective and became part of the team, so to speak. Can you tell me how that unfolded during the week?

(The client is now in hypnosis again)

What has the tiny part communicated to you?

Ah. That is very interesting, as I think you will agree. And how does that tiny part think that the worry could be alleviated?

Oh, I see. How are you going to help that to happen?

(She is in hypnosis again)

First possibility: **The idea worked, and the "tiny part" took on a little role of its own, including some ideas as to how to release some of the free-floating anxiety:**

This could be a concern over past events, for example, and a fear that it would happen again—even though you, or she, may never know how that started.

The tiny part has offered some sort of suggestion regarding this. The important thing is to find a way to utilize that suggestion, whatever it might be.

Whatever the suggestion, find a way to help her get started, reminding her that she has already made a huge step towards healing—and she has done it herself!

Second possibility: **The idea worked, but she feels that there must be more to it. She is concerned about this, and you want to alleviate that anxiety as quickly as possible.**

Yes, there may well be more to be explored. Do you want to do that? (*Yes*) Then ask that wise, subconscious mind of yours to go backwards in time, backwards in time to find or remember some incident that you have forgotten about, at a conscious level, but that is somehow connected with these anxieties. Then you can explore that connection further, using your own self-hypnosis; or we can do that here, now or in future sessions, if you prefer.

The client will almost always discover some incident or more information that she feels offers further explanation of the root cause of her anxiety. Then you and she can go forward with that, with the expectation that it will bring relief.

Panic attacks

As with any anxiety disorder, panic attacks can be in response to a specific situation, or may appear for no apparent reason whatsoever.

Specific situation

If it is in response to a specific situation, then I have found that simple techniques work very well. These would include breathing techniques (which have already been mentioned), relaxation and calming with the help of a code word, and self-reassurance (the story of *The Little Train That Could*).

Tom, you've explained that you still become quite overwhelmed every time you enter the board room for a Directors Meeting. It's really getting you down. Is that right? (*Yes*)

Making sure you're on the same wavelength

Then settle yourself onto hypnosis in your own way, and when you are ready, take yourself into that board room, where there is going to be a meeting in a few minutes. Let me know when you have done that, and knowing at the same time that you are safe here in my office. (*Signals*)

Few people have any trouble with being "present" in two places; if someone does, simply say that it is alright to be in both places

That's right. Now, focus on releasing muscle tension throughout your body in a sequential way, from head to toes, until you feel that the tightness has eased. And as you are doing that, repeat a code word of your own choice, over and over, just silently to yourself. Nobody else needs to know that you are doing this, so you can keep it completely personal.

The "sequential" part is important—the code word itself doesn't matter; it is the repetition that matters. Once chosen, most people keep the same code word

Now that you have established your code word, it is yours to use whenever you need it. Feel the sense of protection in that. Um-hum. Very good.

Post-hypnotic suggestion—"feel the sense of protection ..."

Now you can bring yourself out of hypnosis in your own way.

It is often helpful to repeat this scenario at least once while he is still in your office. Repetition seems to solidify the suggestion.

Another script

Betty, you've told me about a response to specific situations that is really interfering with your life. Your usual techniques aren't working very well. Would you like to explore a different approach? (*Yes*)

Then settle down in your own way, and then take yourself to whatever level of hypnosis seems just right at this time. Let me know when you are at that level. (*After a few moments, signals*)

She will know when she is ready

Good. Do you remember the story about *The Little Train That Could*? (*Nods*) Then think of this story in connection to the aggravation that keeps intruding, and think of eliminating that aggravation, while all the time saying to yourself that little mantra: "I think I can, I think I can, I think ..." and as the aggravation begins to lessen, then change it to: "I can, I can, I can, I can ..." until the sense of intrusion is gone and you can say, "I DID!"

There's nothing like going back to what worked in childhood!

She may be giggling while she is doing this, but since it is working for her, keep at it

Success!

Excellent! Now come out of hypnosis in your own way, knowing that you have found a very easy way to conquer that aggravation, whenever it seems to interfere with what you want to do.

Reaffirmation, focusing on "*you have found ...*" so that she can own that success

"No reason" panic attacks

These come out of the blue and can be extremely debilitating. The person feels completely helpless and is absolutely sure that they are going to die. It happens in ordinary situations like being in a line-up in a grocery store, sitting in a movie theatre or on a crowded bus. While feeling that sense of doom, there is also terrible embarrassment because the need to get away, leave the line or climb over people in the theatre takes precedence over any societal nicety.

When asked what they fear, people will often reply, "Making a fool of myself."

Often establishing a specific routine to follow as soon as the symptoms appear will help. It is a rather obsessive–compulsive remedy, but it works.

Phobias

A phobia, according to the dictionary, is an irrational fear of something (or someone), and a subsequent frantic effort to avoid coming into contact with that object or entity.

Phobias are, in fact, a type of fear response when there is little (in the situation) to fear. There is a difference between being frightened or anxious, and being phobic—the latter being a response out of context with the gravity of the encounter. It is reasonable to be somewhat anxious about a rattlesnake or a man with a gun, but unreasonable—phobic—to be frightened out of one's wits by a garter snake or by seeing any man who happens to wear a slouched hat.

However, as is so often the case, it doesn't matter whether it is reasonable or not to the person who is rigid with fear. The terror is real.

Those who have been in extremely traumatic circumstances may find themselves phobic about any person, object, or circumstance that might bear the slightest resemblance to the traumatic events. Reason has nothing to do with it; it is the connection that is so utterly intrusive.

For some, good cognitive behavioural therapy can work wonders. Others, though, cannot manage that logical shift. This is where hypnosis can help.

Charles, we have talked about the interference that these phobic reactions are causing for you, really intruding into your day-to-day life in many ways. And you are telling me that it seems to be getting worse. Is that correct? (*Yes*)	**Making sure of the problem**
And we have decided to explore using hypnosis, which adds a different dimension to experience. Do you still feel comfortable about doing that? (*Signals "Yes"*)	**Making sure that he is ready**
Alright. Then as you settle yourself into your own hypnosis, arrange the room or the furniture so that you can put up a strong, but almost transparent, curtain between you and what you are going to be watching. Let me know when you have done that. (*In a few moments, signals "Yes"*)	**It is important that he makes the arrangements himself**
Very good. Now, in your own way, allow yourself to see just the smallest corner of a picture that shows (*whatever might relate to the traumatic situation*). Only the smallest corner, remember. And focus on your breathing while you see that tiny corner.	**"The smallest corner" is very important**
Breathe evenly and slowly, knowing that you are safe, here in my office, watching that tiny, tiny corner of the picture. Just continue to do that.	**Controlled breathing gives him something to focus on while he is also focusing on the tiny corner—thus automatically lowering the fear**

(*Allow this to go on for several minutes, as you monitor his breathing and body language, and you continue to make "helpful noises", as Dr Claire Frederick would say. See page 83*)

You are managing this very well, Charles. Now you can allow just the *teeniest* tiny bit more of the picture to be seen.

Continuing the process

You continue in this way, until you feel that he has had enough for that day. Congratulate him on a job well done but still in progress, and make an appointment for him to return in a few days—no longer than a week, in my experience. He can practice this at home, but only if he feels safe in doing that.

When he returns:

Charles, are you ready to explore a little further now? (*Yes*) Excellent. Then take yourself into your hypnosis again, and let me know when you are the level you feel is just right, *this* time.

Getting set again to proceed

(*Nods*) Good. Then once again, bring that corner of the picture into focus, and let me know when you have done that. (*Nods*)

Now, you can either keep adding small pieces to the picture, *or* you can add another layer to the curtain, whichever you feel is best. Let me know when you have done that. (*After a moment, nods*) Thank you.

This is different; he has some options as to how he can protect himself

If he has added another tiny piece to the corner, proceed as before. If he has chosen to add another layer to the curtain, you can say:

Now you can decide to look at as much of the picture as you choose, because you have that extra safety layer of the curtain. And as you look, you will realize that *you are looking at an old picture, <u>not</u> at a current situation.* And that that is different. A picture of something that has happened in the past is different from something that is happening right now.

And this is the crucial shift: you are presenting him with *logic*, and this is the door to a new understanding—that the past is not the present

And you can continue to remember that, any time you need to remember that a picture of the past is different from what is happening in the present.

A tool that he can use himself— another door, toward self-sufficiency

Obviously, this is a contrived situation, but it is representative of the kinds of problems phobic people cope with every day, and offers some possibilities for helping themselves to get out of the mire.

Depression

One of the most intrusive aspects of trauma, especially Post-Traumatic Stress Disorder and related problems, is the depression that often accompanies it. It is not just the "I feel blue today" type of depression; it is the intrusive, overwhelming sense of failure: "what-is-the-use-of-anything," "I'm a blight on society" kind of depression. It erodes all sense of self-worth. Medication may help—and does help some; but not all, and not the deepest, most intrusive types of this desperate disorder. It is an imbalance of brain chemistry, and we need to be aware of that.

As is so often the case with trauma disorders, one must be particularly aware of the potential for doing harm rather than good. That said, one can explore carefully and get a sense of whether or not hypnotic techniques might bring a positive dimension.

Daphne, we've been talking about hypnosis, and discussing whether that might be helpful for you, to counterbalance that depression that you have been battling for some time now. Are you still interested in exploring that? (*Yes*)	**Making sure that she wants to do this**
Alright. Then just settle into hypnosis in the way that you have learned how to do, and use your breathing to release muscle tension. That's it, good. Stay with that for a few more moments.	**Releasing muscle tension is always a good way to start. She begins to feel that she is in charge—something that depression erodes**
Now, begin to find some part of your body that is more comfortable than other parts, and focus on that part for a little while. Find out *why* it is more comfortable. Sometimes it is because it feels just a little lighter, somehow. See if that is part of the awareness for you.	**This is an implied suggestion** **Bolstering the implication** **Hypnotic suggestion**

Presuming that it is, then you can find a way to let that lightness spread through other, nearby, parts of your body, too. Just focus on that for a little time, and let me know when that is happening.

Implicit suggestion that it is, indeed, happening. This adds a sense of power that she can appreciate

And because we know that we are never, never disconnected at the neck, you can understand that your brain is benefiting from this, also.

To utilize the mind–body communication in a positive way; it implies assurance, rather than depression

That's excellent, Daphne. You can understand how mind and body can help each other to feel well, and get well. Now you can let your mind and body be even more in sync, both feeling more positive and more worthy. It's wonderful, isn't it, how we can teach our minds and our bodies to help each other?

The implied suggestion is one of control, rather than feeling out of control

And we know that our brains make some special substances—hormones and biochemicals—to help us maintain that sense of well-being. Talk to your mind and your body together, just for the next few minutes, to strengthen this new knowledge that you have had, but maybe didn't know that you have had for a long time. I'll be quiet while you do that. You can nod when you have had that conversation. (*In a few moments, nods or signals*)

More implied suggestions. Hypnosis utilizes *perception*, not logic

"Hypnospeak"

Very good. In a few moments, then, you can bring yourself out of hypnosis in your own way, bringing all that new understanding with you.

In such situations, it is usually helpful to arrange follow-up sessions fairly soon—within a few days. There is no reason why these hypnotic sessions cannot comfortably co-exist with medication. If so, suggestions that the mind and body can both make the very best possible use of that medication enhance the positive effect. You can use the same format, only changing it in minor ways to reaffirm the message.

Grief and bereavement

Although we often use these words synonymously, they do not really mean the same thing. We can certainly grieve without death being a part of that, and sometimes death brings a softer grief than at other times. What may bring unrelenting grief to one person may present only a short-term sense of absence, and perhaps some disappointment, in another.

The following is a somewhat simplistic script for a young woman—perhaps even a teenager—whose friend has moved away. You can use it as a model which you can expand to suit the particular situation.

Jennie, you've told me that you are feeling very sad about the loss of your friend, because he has moved to another city. Would you like to talk some more about that? (*No, there's nothing I can do about it*)	**Opening the interaction**
That's true, so perhaps you would like to explore another way of letting go of the sense of loss. We talked about some hypnosis. Shall we explore that? (*Yes*) Alright. Then just settle yourself down, as you did a few weeks ago when we were practicing this technique. (*After a few moments, settles in*)	**At least, it's something different**
That's right. And pay attention to the tension in your body, and breathe it away, as you learned how to do last time we practiced this. That's right, just breathe the tension away. I can see your muscles relaxing.	**Releasing muscle tension is always helpful**
(*A little time passes—only a minute or two by clock time*) You are doing that very well, Jennie.	**Positive reinforcement**

Now you can begin to remember good times that you had with your friend, and think about how happy you are that you have those memories. It would be sad to be left without those memories, wouldn't it? (*Yes*) Yes, it would be. So maybe you could put those memories in a special place, like putting pictures in a photograph album. Or you could do both; then you would have a real book of memories and also another book of very happy times, in your imagination memory. Just take a few minutes now and explore some of the possibilities. Let me know when you have decided how you are going to do that. (*After a few moments, nods*) That's very good, Jennie. And I can see that you have a little less tension in your face and body now. So it helps, doesn't it, to have a new way of remembering those good times? And as you know, you can have those comforting memories and thoughts for as long as you wish. (*She sighs, and nods*)

Shifting the scene toward being happy with memories, instead of having nothing

How to utilize this

Yet another possibility

Reassurance and pinpointing the positive effects

Although this script is aimed more at younger people, it can of course be adapted for anyone. We all tend to go back to our memories of childhood when we are unhappy.

For the loss of a loved one through death, there is very often a series of emotional responses that are typical of grieving or bereavement. We know that they will not be coming back, but there is still a denial of the fact. This denial is very, very common, even when the death was expected or partially expected. It is as if our worst fear has come true. People often feel a sense of anger—even fury—and then of numbness.

Denial and anger are often followed by bargaining: "If only he'll come back I'll do anything …" Of course, he is not going to come back and then the facts must be faced. At that time, anger often comes forward, with thoughts or even shouts of, "It's not fair! How dare he leave me like that? I'm not ready for this!" often followed by weeping. This anger comes and goes, often in unexpected moments. It may be directed at anyone, even those (sometimes especially those) who have cared for the person who has died—doctors, nurses, other family members.

There may be, and often is, a sense of yearning so intense as to be almost insupportable. People wonder, "How am I ever going to get through this?" And then there is the dreadful sensation of guilt: "What did I do? Where did I go wrong?" In cases of severe trauma, such as war, those in command often feel guilty and angry at the same time. This is often a major part of Post-Traumatic Stress Disorder.

Depression may follow, then hollowness, and finally, acceptance.

The work of Dr Elisabeth Kübler-Ross has been recognized as a working pattern to help get people through grief and bereavement. They are: denial, anger, bargaining, depression, acceptance. Although the sequence is never cut and dried, the pattern has proven to be generally representative of what happens.

Harry, you miss her dreadfully, so much so that you are making yourself ill. The medication isn't helping. Would you agree to do some hypnosis? (*I guess so, if you want to*) Let's see if it can be helpful. If it is, that will be good. If not, we don't have to do it again. Is that alright? (*Yes*)

Recognizing the need for more specific work

Make yourself comfortable, then, and let your eyes close when you are ready. As you are settling in, focus on your breathing, slow and steady, to keep *you* steady. That's right.

As is so often the case, the breathing pattern takes the mind off the main issue for a few moments, which breaks the intensity

The way you are feeling—although of course it is very personal—is similar to what most people feel when they lose someone they love. But there are some things that you can always keep: memories of her face, her laughter, her hair, her voice, her body, her essence. These are things that you can have, always. Take a little time now, to remember her in those ways.

Reassurance that he is not alone in experiencing this

Changing the perspective

Tears may begin to roll down his face. You can gently offer him a tissue, but he may not wish to take it.

And the love that you shared will never go away. It will always be there, inside you, whatever the future may hold.

At times, people wonder whether they are being disloyal, if the sorrow abates, even just a little bit

(*This is true, even if he decides to re-marry; it need not impose on the new relationship, because it has a special place in the <u>old</u> relationship. But that is for the future.*)

Now find, within yourself, a very special place for her. A *very, very* special place, and she can always be there, for you. You can visit her whenever you like, and you will find, in time, that the love takes over the sadness. So you can be patient, knowing that that happens.

This relieves the concern over disloyalty and offers hope that the desperate sense of loss will ease

You can always use your self-hypnosis, too, to give yourself a little space when you need it. It is comforting to know that you can do that.

Helping to establish that *he* can do that himself

We seldom give much thought to the emotional turmoil many women face when they have decided to have a therapeutic abortion. This is often accompanied by a sense of social distain—although that has lessened in the past few decades. This script has its origins in my recounting a story to a woman in my family practice, many years ago, who had had a therapeutic abortion years before. I told her about my experience in Japan while visiting a beautiful park that was a memorial park for infants that had been aborted, and the peace that this offered to the women who had had to make that decision.

Angela, you have been thinking about the situation I discovered while I was in Japan. Would you like to explore that again in hypnosis? (*Yes*)

Setting the scene

Yes, I think so, too. So settle into your hypnosis, as you know how to do, and let me know when you have reached the level that seems right for you at this time. (*After a little time, signals*)

That's right. Now you can take yourself, in your own way and in your own thoughts, to a little memorial park similar to the one I described for you last week. And you can spend a little time in that lovely place—as long as you like in hypnosis time, while I watch the clock time for you, to discover what you need to discover. (*Two or three minutes by clock time*) Would you like to be there a little longer? (*If yes, do that*)

Making the memorial park more of a reality for her, personally

The time is personal for each client

(*When ready*) That's right. I can see that you have found some sense of comfort. Is that right? (*Yes*) Good. You can keep that, and call on it any time you need to do so. And perhaps you have decided on something you want to do, also (*I do not wait for an answer here, as she can make that decision herself, now or at a later time if she wishes*) When you are ready, then, you can bring yourself out of hypnosis in your own way.

In a way, this is giving her permission to something that would bring some degree of comfort

Quite often, women will choose to make a little memorial in their own garden, or at a beach. This has proven to be extremely helpful; the grieving eases and healing begins, sometimes years after the abortion occurred.

A similar approach can be made in the case of stillbirths, although the sense of guilt may not be there, or at least not so intensely.

Children

Children also need help, when someone in the family or a very special friend is dying or has died. For many, it is a dilemma, to know how to tell them, and yet they need to know.

A gentle hypnosis approach can sometimes be helpful.

Debbie, I know that your grandmother has died. I think that maybe you are feeling very upset and confused about that. Is that true? (*"Yes"*)

Clarifying the situation

Did you get a chance to say goodbye to her? (*No—maybe some tears*) That's alright, you can cry if you want. But I think that I know something that can help you to feel better. Would you like that? (*Nods*)

It's important to bring the situation back into normalcy

Alright. Then just sit back in that comfy chair and close your eyes. That's right. And now pretend that you and your grandma are talking. Can you do that? (*Nods*) Good.

Children go into hypnosis at the drop of a hat

You can tell her about your day, what you have been doing, and the things that you and she used to talk about. Yes, that's right. (*She is obviously talking to her grandmother*)

Again, getting back to normal things

That's a very good conversation you are having. And it's almost time to finish that conversation now, so tell her anything more that you need to tell her. (*Obviously this is happening*)

Reassurance and giving her time to finish what she is saying

Yes, that was a good conversation. And now it's time for you to say goodbye to her, because she isn't very well and she's very tired. She needs to go to a place where she is safe. We call that "dying". It's a nice, peaceful place. But it's important for you to say goodbye, and so can she, so you can do that now. (*She says goodbye*)

And time to say goodbye

Reassurance that Grandma isn't hurting any more

And when you are ready, in a minute or so, you can open your eyes again. That's right. Your Mummy is out there in the waiting room. Do you want to go to her now? (*Yes*) Okay. Maybe I'll see you in a few days—will that be alright? (*Yes*)

Leaving the door open for a further session if necessary

Palliative care

Family members who have a dear relative or very special friend in palliative care, often feel that "There must be something I can *do*..." even though what has needed to be done, has been done. Palliative care centres are very special, with highly trained staff. They are the ones taking medical and nursing care of the client, and they do it superbly well. What we can do is visit, send cards, bring pictures (*very* important for some people) talk about day-to-day things—whatever the one being cared for would like to hear or see.

If that person is close to dying, then it is often important for those closest to them to give them permission to go. It can be as simple as saying, "It's alright, dear; you can go when you're ready." A sigh, a nod, a smile on the loved one's face will let us know that that is the case, that is what they have been waiting for and needed to hear.

Although this is not specific hypnosis, people very near the end of their lives are often already in an altered state of consciousness and perceive messages in that mental/emotional milieu.

Many years ago, I had a woman client, quite young, who was dying from a miserable, implacable disease. She had a loving husband and two children, one in her teens, another a few years younger.

She had just returned from one of the major clinics in the United States; nothing more could be done. She was supposed to come in for a hypnosis session, but her husband phoned to say that she was in the palliative care ward at our local hospital. I went up to see her after office hours, and she was a clearly anxious, so agreed quickly to some hypnosis. I just did a basic, soothing hypnosis, and at the end of it I told her that she could stay in hypnosis, or fall asleep, or waken, which ever she chose. It soon became obvious that she was going to stay in her hypnosis, and I thought that she would probably drift from there into sleep, which is what happened. Before I left, I said that I would see her in the morning. There was a slight nod—she had heard me.

When I arrived the next morning, the nurses told me that they thought that they had lost her several times during the night, but then she had started to breathe again.

I walked into her room. She looked to be asleep. I greeted her—"Good morning, Julia." (*For obvious reasons, that was not her name but the one I have chosen to call her here.*)

She opened her eyes, smiled at me and said "Good morning, Dr. Hunter", and peacefully died. She had waited for me, it seemed, as she had indicated that she would. I will never forget her, or that moment.

Section III

Dissociative Disorders

Important: The use of hypnosis when working with clients who have a Dissociative Disorder should only be done when the therapist is well-trained in both the psychotherapy for dissociation (as a disorder) and in the use of hypnosis with this client population. This section presumes that the therapist is educated and experienced in both these regards.

Safety—inside and out

Psychotherapy always demands attention to safety and containment, both emotional and physical. Never is this more important than when working with someone who suffered abuse as a child. The issue of keeping oneself safe, therefore, is first and foremost on the agenda.

And because people who have been abused as a child are often reluctant to go into hypnosis—it being too reminiscent of the state they were in during the abuse—it behooves us to give this aspect the attention it deserves, and describe hypnosis, its uses and opportunities, and its possible effects, clearly.

This first script presumes that the client has already done some hypnosis and is comfortable with it.

First script

Alison, now that you are comfortably in hypnosis, at whatever level you know is just right for you *this* time, pause and take a look around you. Although you know that you are in my office, or that you are safely at home, you can use that knowledge to help you when you are feeling worried or distressed or scared.

Using the usual hypnotic technique that she is used to, let her get settled down comfortably, taking whatever time it needs

Reassure her that she knows how to do this herself

You know that you can, if and when you choose, take yourself to one of those safe places again—perhaps feeling yourself to be in my office, or perhaps transposing yourself to somewhere that's a special place at home—a room that is warm and comfortable, or that has some very happy memories. Or some other very, very safe place, that you know feels right for you.	**It is up to her—she has the control** **Offer several familiar choices**
Let yourself feel that safety, that security that comes from knowing that you are in a safe place.	**Experience the sense of security**
And reassure yourself, over and over again, you can do that, you can go to that safe place, any time *you* choose, no matter what else may be going on around you.	**Continuing reassurance that she has the control, *no matter whatever else may be going on around her***
And you can stay in that safe place for as long as you choose. It is *your* decision.	

Second script

N.B. This script presumes that the psychotherapy uses the ego-state approach. For other approaches, the therapist can modify the script to suit the situation.

The client has been invited to go into hypnosis in their own way, similar to the beginning of the above script.

Now, because you know how important it is for you to *know* that you are safe both inside and out, look round you very carefully, in your hypnosis, and make sure that, in your hypnosis, you are very safe on the *outside*.	**Establishing the importance of a very safe place to go to, when it is necessary** **When the client is in the world, so to speak—e.g. at work**
Then, when you have made very, very sure that you are safe on the outside, begin to look around on the inside.	
Look carefully, and see how safe it is for you on the inside.	**Being safe inside is often a greater challenge because of the structure of the personality**

Can you see and know that all parts of you are safe? Every single part?

Look very carefully for the children. Are they all in a very safe place? Do they all have an older part to take care of them? Do they look comfortable and at ease?

Feeling safe is very individual, and child ego states are particularly vulnerable

If any of them look the least little bit uncomfortable, take time to find out why, before you go any further.

It is acceptable for the therapist to advise in this situation, if it seems appropriate

Often, child parts enjoy being in a group together. They may want to play a game.

This is also a preliminary step towards *blending*, which is described on page 140

Adult parts, too, need to know that they are very safe inside. Look at and talk to each part, specifically, and make sure that it is safe for each one of them.

Adults are vulnerable, too

As you know, they may have a special place where they like to go—a garden, the seashore, a comfortable room. Help them to get to their most comfortable place. Do they need to have a wall or fence to feel more secure? Be sure that they have a key to the gate, if there is a wall, and that the gate is locked behind them.

The therapist is acknowledging the important role of the client themselves in this endeavour. This improves the sense of self worth, which is almost always lacking in trauma survivors

Take your time, because it is important.

Once you *all* know that you are safe and secure, just relax and enjoy being where you are. And know that you can all go there, whenever you choose and whenever you need to.

Again stressing the important active role of the client

This safe place belongs to *you*, only you, and nobody else can come in, unless you allow them to do so. If you allow anybody else in, be very sure that the person you allow in is a very safe person, too.

Reinforcing the above

You can go there individually, also, if any part of you wants or needs to do that.

Often it helps if there is a special word
that you can say to yourself, to help you
get to that special place quickly. We call it
a "code word". You may want to choose
a code word right now, so that you will
have it whenever you might need it. The
code word can be very private, so that
nobody on the outside knows what it is,
or you may choose to tell a special person
what it is. That choice is up to you—only
to you.

Code words are very useful in stressful situations when a more thought-out process is difficult

Always let the client choose the code word. It improves the sense of "I can do it" (again, this can strengthen self-worth)

Take as long as you like, now, in hypnosis
time, to be in that special, safe place. I'll
watch the time for you, and let you know
how the clock time is passing.

This is an old and ever-useful ploy to invite the client to tidy up any unfinished odds and ends from the hypnosis session.

(Therapist advises the client of the clock time: "Now half of the clock time has passed …" "Now three-quarters if the clock time has passed …" etc.)

It will soon be time to come out of your
hypnosis for today. Of course, you can do
this at home any time you choose, or use
your code word if you need to get there
quickly, but in an eyes-open hypnosis. Use
hypnosis, whenever it might be important
for you to do that.

Further reassurance—"*you* can do this yourself, any time you need to or want to." It may be useful to have the client practice this in the safety of your office

Then invite the client to come out of hypnosis in their own way.

Helping the child part to tell

Often when working through past traumata, and when there is significant
dissociativity, one part of the personality structure believes that they know
more than other parts. And very often, the part that knows is a young
child. However, that child part may not have the understanding or experience to be able to describe what they know. In such a situation, hypnosis
can play a very helpful role.

We also need to be aware that children perceive situations differently to
adults, because as children, our interpretations are based on perception
rather than logic. We know that this person, as a child, was subjected
to trauma—emotional, physical or sexual, or some combination of the

three—and that her interpretation of the events will be remembered in that context: fear, pain, confusion, abandonment.

The client has agreed that hypnosis could be helpful and is settling into a comfortable chair. Note that the agreement of the client is essential.

I'm speaking now to all parts of Susan. Some of you are older and some younger, but Little Susan has told us that she has something that she knows about, but is afraid to tell us. Who can help Little Susan to tell us?

Establishing the scene, and that everyone is participating

Further clarification as to what the conversation is to be about, and that Little Susan needs help

(Take time for the various parts to discuss this, and come to a conclusion)

Very important to allow time to agree on the situation

Ah, Jennifer is going to help Little Susan. That's excellent. But first of all, let's be sure that everybody is comfortable.

The various ego states have made a decision, indicating that they are collaborating

That's right. Good.

Comfort level also established

Jennifer, perhaps you can reassure Little Susan that she is safe, here in my office, and you are with her, close to her, so that she can reach out and touch you if she wishes. Can you do that? Good.

Again confirming comfort level and safety—very important

Utilizing touch sensation between the ego states

Now Little Susan, would it be easier for you to tell Jennifer rather than to tell me? Because you know her much better than you know me, right? Of course you do, and that's easy to understand.

Validating the decision to tell another part rather than to tell me, which could be perceived as dangerous

So you tell Jennifer about something that happened, and you feel very upset about it. Maybe you were hurt, or very scared. You can whisper to her, if it is easier for you to do that, and then Jennifer can tell me.

Allowing time for communication to occur

Understanding the child part's hesitancy about disclosing

(At this point, Little Susan may become very distressed that Jennifer is going to tell me, because then Susan could be accused of breaking her promise to "never tell", or bad things would happen to her, or to someone else.)

Jennifer, Little Susan may be upset. Take a minute to reassure her that it is safe, now, to tell you about what happened. That's right. Is she more comfortable now? Good.	**Affirming that the perceived fear is real to the child part and that it is safe, because she is going to tell Jennifer, not me (i.e. "keep it in the family", so to speak)**
That's right. I can see that Little Susan is whispering to Jennifer. She can take as long as she needs to tell what she needs to tell. Jennifer, you can nod to me when Little Susan has finished telling you what she needs to tell you.	**There is no rush, it is important to be able to tell it calmly**

Time always becomes distorted in hypnosis, so if it seems that the "telling" is going to take longer than is realistic, the therapist can make a comment such as "Take as long as you need in hypnosis time, and I'll watch the clock time for you", and then at suitable intervals—such as twenty seconds or so—mention that "half the clock time is over now" or similar comments to keep things on track. This works amazingly well in most situations.

Ahh. There is a little nod. Jennifer, has she been able to tell you what she needed to tell you? (*Jennifer signals, yes*) Good.	**Watch carefully, so that you do catch the signal, which may be minimal**
Little Susan, you are a very brave girl. Is there more that you need to tell Jennifer right now?	**Validating Little Susan's courage** **Look for a nod or head shake**

If it is a shake of the head, then close the hypnosis. If it is a nod, set a time limit such as, "Alright, take another minute or so by clock time, and I'll let Jennifer know how the time is passing."

Remember that this may seem minor to the therapist, but gut-wrenching to the client so give the client a minute or so to collect herself. Then gently ask:

Can you tell me about it now? We have some time left in the session.	**Offering the opportunity to share the new knowledge and begin to put it into perspective**

After a disclosure

After a disclosure to the therapist, the client may be anxious that they may have done a bad thing in disclosing and/or be afraid of retribution. Although this may seem unlikely or nonsensical to the therapist, it may be very real to the client and needs to be treated with the greatest respect. If there is considerable anxiety, a brief hypnotic intervention may be useful.

The client has agreed that there is anxiety regarding a recent disclosure and that a short hypnotic session may be useful in dispelling that anxiety. The hypnosis has just begun and the client is resting but may still be obviously tense.

Jennifer, you have been feeling some anxiety after last week's session, is that right? (*Nods or signals "yes"*)	**Defining the situation**
But I think that also it brought some new clarification or understanding, is that right also? (*Nods or signals "yes" again*)	**Reassuring that something positive was happening**
Um-hum, I understand.	**Further reassurance**
It was an important disclosure, was it not? With very important information? Because that is what made the information so important—so that everybody could know something that they may not have known before.	**Validating the importance of what happened—the client may not have put it in that perspective**
Is it that Little Susan is upset or afraid? Or that you or others are afraid?	**Making sure you know exactly where the agitation resides**
Then every part of you needs to feel very proud that Little Susan was brave enough to describe how she felt.	**Knowing your client, you may choose to say "can feel" rather than "needs to feel"**
Just take a few moments now, to enjoy that new feeling of being very proud. You and all parts of you deserve to enjoy that feeling.	**Putting it into a different perspective—something to be proud of**
So now you can know that you have done something very good indeed, and that it will help you as you get well.	**Reaffirming the positive and relieving anxiety of disclosing**

A very simple reassuring technique is for the client—in or out of hypnosis—to find the most comfortable place in their body at that time and, through breathing, draw the comfortable feelings in while breathing in, and then send them throughout the whole body as they breathe out. Several deep breaths can accomplish this, along with the suggestion that it is, indeed, a very simple method which can be used any time, any place, in any circumstance. "After all, everybody <u>breathes</u>!"

Alternative technique

Another useful gimmick to help the child part to tell is for them to "tell" a favorite toy, e.g. a cuddly teddy bear. Bear in mind that the child is in an adult body, so the therapist must feel comfortable with this also. Fewer male clients will respond to this technique than female clients, so there is another script for male clients following this one.

So, Jennifer, I understand that the Little One has something that she feels she must tell, but she doesn't know how to do that, because she is afraid. Is that right?	**Setting the agenda; establishing the situation and how it can be handled**
Um-hum. So we must find a way for her to tell, but still feel safe. Is that right? (*She nods her head or signals with her fingers*)	**Reassuring safety**
Then if that is how she will feel safe, we must, of course, do as she asks. I am wondering if she would feel safe holding Teddy, and telling him? Could you ask her about that?	**Respectful to the client and to all her parts** **Suggesting a solution**
(*Give her a few seconds and watch for an ideomotor response, such as a nod.*)	
Ah. That's it, then. Here you are, Little One—your favourite Teddy. (*Child part reaches out, takes the Teddy and clearly feels more comfortable*)	**It needs to be a Teddy that she has seen and cuddled before**
Very good. Now, Little One, you tell Teddy what you need to tell him and let Jennifer and me know when you have finished telling. Is that alright? (*Nods*) Good.	**Reassurance that now it is safe to tell Teddy, so that Teddy can then tell Jennifer or me. This is important, because the child part could feel betrayed if it is not clarified first**

At this point, the therapist settles back and, watching closely, lets it happen. The motor movements, mouthing and facial appearance will all let the therapist know how things are going. If it goes on too long, then gently suggest that it is wonderful that she has almost finished telling Teddy what she needs to tell.

That was very good and brave of you, Little One. But then, we know that Teddy is a safe person to tell, isn't that right? (*Nods*) And then Teddy can tell Jennifer, or me, what *we* need to know, when you are safely tucked away inside and nobody can hurt you. (*Nods*)

Reassuring and praising her and emphasizing again that Teddy is safe

Reiterating the next step

Good. So you can rest now, and I'll talk to Jennifer and Teddy.

Praise for a job well done

Script modified for male client

Don, there is a technique that works well when there is a child part inside who has knowledge but is afraid to tell for fear of reprisal. Often we do this in hypnosis, but we can do it without hypnosis— whichever feels more comfortable for you.

Establishing the scene and its format

The technique is the same, in or out of hypnosis—the client will probably go into an altered state anyway

Of course, you are aware of Young Don and the role he plays. He seems to be one of the Keepers of Secrets, is that right? And it also seems that he is in need of telling about some past experience now, but doesn't know how to do that, or is fearful, as we have said.

Verifying the Keeper of Secrets and the fact that he needs to tell someone, but that someone must be very safe

So I'm wondering if he would like to go up in his favourite rocket, and then he could tell The Commander, and he would be safe because they will be out in space. Could you ask him about that? (*Watch the ideomotor responses—nodding of the head, etc.*)

This conversation presumes that Young Don is listening, as he is almost bound to be

Good. So, Young Don, would you like to go out in space and find out what's going on in that Other World? And while you are there, you can tell The Commander what it is that you need to tell. How does that sound? Because you will be out in space and therefore very safe from Earth-Aliens.

Making it more personal, now, with Young Don

Because *no one* is as safe as The Commander

In other words, people who could hurt you

(*Vigorous nodding from Young Don*)

Excellent. Take off then, as you know how
to do, and have a great journey.

**Leaving it up to him now,
because he knows how to do it**

*Watch carefully, so you will know when he has fulfilled his need to tell The
Commander and is ready to come back to earth.*

When you are ready, then, Young
Don, come back to earth and into this
room. Very good. Did you have a good
flight? And were you able to tell The
Commander what you needed to tell him?

**Bringing him back into the
present room and situation, i.e.
he is in your office**

Make sure that it happened!

Very good. And now he can take care of
it, can't he? Because that's part of his job.
(*Watch for the relieved nods*)

**It is important to stress that it is,
indeed, part of his job**

*Make the appropriate closing comments and reassure your client that he has done
very well. You may wish to finish the session now, or go on to something else.
Usually it is helpful to avoid questioning regarding "Did it work?" We presume
that it <u>did</u> work, and that at the next session, he will have something to discuss
with you.*

Safety shields when working through the trauma
Establishing various sorts of safety shields, using hypnotic techniques,
offers yet another level of security for an abuse survivor when working
through their traumatic experiences.

Jane, you've decided that you are ready to
work through one of those memories that
has been plaguing you for so long. Do you
still feel ready to do that today? (*Nods*)

**It is important to establish
that she is ready—sometimes
the client is reluctant to admit
that she has changed her mind,
because she is afraid that you
might think less of her, or that
some of her parts might call her
a wimp**

Then just settle yourself into a very secure
level of hypnosis, as you know how to do.
Let me know when you have reached that
level of security. (*In time, she nods*)

**Note: If she is not ready, tell her
that you appreciate her telling
you that, and she can tell you in
her own time, when she *is* ready**

Good. Now you know how important it is to keep safe, and one excellent way to keep safe through hypnosis is to create a safety shield around yourself. In fact, you can create *two* safety shields, one for emotional distress and then another one for physical and sexual distress. Let's start with the emotional distress: Is that a good thing to do first? (*Nods*) Yes, it is.

The concept of an hypnotic shield is both practical and imaginative, and therefore appeals to both the perceptual parts of the mind and to the logical parts of the mind. There is *always* emotional trauma, whether or not there has been physical and/or sexual trauma

It is important to establish the shield in whatever way seems just right for you. Many people wrap themselves in an invisible blanket, one that is impermeable to every emotional onslaught. But it important for you to do it in your own way. Let me know when you are ready for the next shield. (*She nods to let you know*)

People usually know what kind of shield suits them best

If we describe it for them, or make a suggestion, it becomes a second-hand shield, which is not what they need

That was very well done. Take another moment or two of hypnosis time to be *absolutely* sure that the shield is impermeable. Let me know that you are ready.

Extra safety, in case there has been some interference from a saboteur

Now, the next shield may need to be of a different type because it is the shield against physical or sexual abuse. You will know the best kind of shield—one especially designed to meet your own personal needs. So you go ahead with that, and let me know, again, when you absolutely know that you have the shield in place. (*She signals*)

Because emotional trauma has a different composition than sexual or physical trauma, it is very important to have specific shields for each of the three trauma components

Now, with those two excellent shields in place, and knowing also that you're in a very safe place, here in my office, you can begin to do whatever you need to do in order to finally put that one—that *one* particular experience—to rest.

Emphasizing, again, the security of your office; *she is not* back at the site of the trauma itself

You know that I am here, and will stay with you while you do that, sending you all my support as you do what you need to do.

Sending support, but not doing it for her; you can make "helpful noises" if and when appropriate

When she has given you a signal that she has finished doing what she needed to do to ameliorate this particular trauma, you can close the session. At times, the client will deal with several traumas in the same session, either as a whole package or one at a time, when there are similarities (as there usually are).

Working through the trauma—in the audience

Another technique that provides emotional security when working through the trauma is to put the traumatic event on a stage, or some equivalent, so that the client can watch it from a distance. Of course, there are many ways to do this; the following offers one suggestion, which can be modified in many ways to suit the individual client.

Carol, you have thought about confronting some of the old traumas and feel that it may be possible to begin to do that. Do you still feel that way? (*Nods*) And you are feeling strong enough to begin to do that today? (*Nods again*) Then we'll begin.

Making sure that she is ready for the work; however, watch your vocal inflection—she would be anxious at any indication that *you* do not think that she is ready

(Note: her nod is equivalent to a commitment to do the work.)

Settle yourself into hypnosis in your own way, to a level that will keep you comfortable today.

She needs to find her own level

Now, imagine that you are in a theatre—a live theatre, rather than a movie. You are in the audience, waiting for the action to begin. Settle into your seat—a seat that is just right, with a good view of the stage. Are you there? (*Nods*) Good. Let the play begin. Describe, for me, what is happening.

Putting distance between herself and the situation—she becomes an observer, not a victim; it is advisable for the therapist to know what is going on in order to intervene, if necessary

She begins to describe the action that is going on "on stage". Limit your responses to the usual "um-hum's" unless you feel that it would be good for her to clarify something. (That might make it easier for you, too!) Absolutely refrain from asking leading questions, such as "Is there anybody else there?"—which indicates that there might be, and may prompt a belief that somehow she needs to find that person.

You have done an excellent job of seeing and describing that scene. And you can now understand it better, too, after putting it into words. Is that what it seems like to you, too? (*Nods*)

Confirming that she has done a good job, to allow her to get on with her life, because she has put the experience into words, transferring some of the emotion from the purely perceptual into the cognitive, and thus diminishing the emotional impact

That's good. You look a little more relaxed, too, so keep that feeling. And, as soon as you are ready, bring yourself out of hypnosis in your own way.

She may need to do some debriefing after this "re-viewing" of the situation. She can do it now, or when she feels more comfortable later. Ask her which she prefers.

Ego strengthening

Applying for a job, writing an exam, etc.

The client has progressed to the point where they are about to undertake a new direction—getting back into the workforce, going back to school, etc. This can be demanding enough at the best of times, but for a person who has been undergoing a difficult psychotherapy for some time, often more than a year or even two, it can be terrifying.

Besides the demand of the job/course/training itself, there is the added stress of returning to the workforce or educational situation.

These scripts presume that the therapist has talked through the positives and not-so-positives of the situation and the client has shown determination to begin this part of the healing process. It is a major step forward, and deserves commendation.

These approaches can be used in or out of hypnosis, whichever is most comfortable for the person involved. And again, as is so often the case, even for those who decide or prefer to do it without hypnosis, a narrowing of focus is almost sure to occur. What is going on in the outside world—which may include your office—is totally outside of their interest at that time.

So Janice, the big day is approaching. And, like everybody in these situations, you are a little anxious—is that right? So today we'll work on relieving the anxiety. Usually we do this exercise in hypnosis, but you can choose whether you want to go into hypnosis or not.	**Setting the scene, neutralizing the anxiety as being normal in such situations** **As always, the client's choice**
Ah. You want to do it in hypnosis. Let yourself get settled in, then, in your own way, as you know how to do.	**She has already had experience of being in hypnosis, and can do her own induction, which offers a sense of empowerment**
Now, spend a few minutes of clock time, but as long as you wish in hypnosis time, to think about the exciting time ahead in the most positive way. After all, this was *your* decision, and you deserve to feel proud about it. Nod when you have given yourself that well-deserved accolade. (*She nods*) Oh, very good indeed. You do deserve to enjoy that positive feeling.	**Beginning to get into the "future–present"** **Important to reinforce that it was her decision, and good one**
Take yourself forward in time, now, and find the day in the future when you are ready to begin this wonderful adventure. *Be* there, in that future time—be present in the future. That's right. Look around you and assure yourself that you are really there, in that future–present. Feel all the feelings, see all there is to see, hear all there is to hear.	**Going into that "future–present" does not seem bizarre to someone in hypnosis** **The sensory aspect is always very important**
You may surprise yourself and find that it is not so scary after all! Ah, yes, I see you smiling a bit. How very nice!	**Helping her to normalize the experience and the anxiety, too**
(*Or: Ah, yes, I see a little anxious look, so you can just <u>breathe</u> and feel more settled. That's right.*)	**Reassuring that these feelings are normal *and* that she has the control**
Now comes the part that's even more interesting. Are you ready? Good! So, take yourself forward even further in time, to the time when you have successfully accomplished what you set out to do. You have that job! (*or, e.g. are enrolled in class*)	**Furthering the experience of time warp to the successful conclusion**

Oh, just really, really enjoy that! Feel so very proud of yourself, as you deserve to be, because you have taken yourself to that positive place, through your own effort and determination. Just enjoy that a little longer.

Further reinforcement of her own accomplishment

Now, slowly bring yourself backwards in time again, towards the *present*–present asking that wise subconscious mind of yours to recognize the signposts along the way. Then, when you make that journey chronologically, your subconscious can recognize the signposts, and keep you on the right path.

Time to return to the "normal" present, and at the same time, to activate the subconscious in a very definitive way

Rationalizing the need for the subconscious awareness (which, of course, is there anyway)

Let me know when you are back in the present–present, secure in my office.

Awareness of where she really is and that she is safe

(*She nods*) Good. Now bring yourself out of hypnosis in your own way.

Closing the hypnosis herself (again offering ego strength)

Speaking up for yourself

Many people who have suffered trauma during childhood, and as a result have developed a dissociative personality structure, are wary of speaking up for themselves. It is true that there is often a part of them which fulfills this function, but all too often that part comes across not as a strong person speaking up for themselves, but instead as rather overbearing and antagonistic, if not downright angry.

It is useful, therefore, to teach some techniques which encourage self-worth, and therefore a capacity to speak politely but assertively in any situation which requires that approach. Hypnosis can be useful in this regard.

Deborah, we've talked several times, in the past few weeks, about learning how to speak up for yourself in a strong but still polite way. Are you interested in doing some of that work now?

Making sure, before starting the hypnosis, that she is still interested in doing this. It must be *her* wish to do so

(*She responds, "Yes, I want to do it."*)

Wait for her affirming response

Alright, then. As we decided last week, one of the most useful techniques is to use hypnosis. Would you like to do that now? (*Nods*) Good. Then take yourself into your hypnosis in your own way, and nod when you have reached the level that seems just right for this task today.

Reminding her of last week's decision

Let me know when you feel that you are at the right level for this work. (*Nods*)

She has the control of the hypnosis

She is still in control

Now, who inside is the best part to do this work? We have talked about several possibilities in the past. Have you decided? (*Nods and answers, "Debbie"*)

This is an important decision, that has already been discussed at some level

Debbie—of course; she is good at things like that, isn't she? So Debbie, come and join Deborah while we talk strategy. Are you happy to do that? (*Nods*)

Confirming the good decision, and getting Debbie to *join* Deborah, thereby encouraging co-conscious interaction

Both of you, think of a recent situation that you wish you had handled better than you did. You can compare notes, because you are in this together, although Debbie is going to be the one to meet with other people when some firm diplomacy is the order of the day. Do you both agree with that way of managing things?

Again, co-conscious action is best to really clarify the boundaries, and to understand the implication of Debbie's role

That's very good. We all have a variety of talents, and in some situations we are better at utilizing them than at other times.

This kind of comment will also re-affirm that we all have ego-states, although some of us have less separation between them

Then think of a situation that happened fairly recently, that you were not really happy about—something that had to do with asserting yourself. Let me know when you have thought of something. (*Nods*)

Letting her set the scene herself, so that she can be comfortable with it

Very good. Do you want to tell me what it was, or would you prefer to keep it private? (*She prefers to keep it private*) Alright, that's fine. Then think of that situation as if it were actually happening again, but do it as if you were yourself offering an opinion as to how you could be doing it better—a sort of running commentary.

Offering the alternative—her choice

Reviewing from a different perspective; *not* **a put-down, just a different perspective**

When you have had a chance to review it, find the areas where you might change something—tone of voice, body language, the wording, or even the place where you decided to speak up.

Offering several possibilities of positive change

I think that you are beginning to see some possibilities. So now you could think about it in a different way—imagining yourself using your improved approach. Find out how that could make the situation less stressful, both for you and for the other person. Let me know when you have had a chance to review it that way. (*Nods*)

Opportunity to practice a new approach

Helpful for both sides

Good—very good indeed. And you see how you have yourself felt stronger by being assertive, but also respectful and not aggressive. Does that feel good? (*Nods*) Yes. So stay in hypnosis for a few more minutes by hypnosis time, then just bring yourself back into this room in your own way, comfortably and confidently.

Offering the opportunity to perceive her ego strength—important

She's in control

After this session, it is important to talk about what happened if the client agrees—it gives her an opportunity to discover an inner strength she didn't realize that she had, <u>without</u> having to look outside herself for help.

Applying for a job

You have discussed with your client the fact that she has decided to apply for a job. It is not a high-powered job, but it is one that will help her to find her feet again in the workforce. She is excited, but also obviously worried that she will make some horrible flub.

It is very courageous of you to go for this interview, so I know that you want to make the best pitch that you can. Are you sure that this job is going to be worth the effort? (*Nods*)	**Encouraging, and adding to her sense of empowerment, while at that same time offering the choice to opt out if she isn't quite ready**
That's good. So we are going to focus on giving a good presentation. Is that right? (*Nods again*) Excellent. Then let us just consider some of the positive things that are part of a good interview. So settle yourself even more comfortably into the level of hypnosis that is just right for you, *this* time. Let me know when you have reached that level. (*Signals*)	**Setting the focus on the scene and beginning to narrow it down to the essential aspects** **Very important for her to feel that she is in her safe level of hypnosis**
There are three important factors which are important in such an interview. One is to stay *calm*. Just think about that for a minute—staying *calm*.	**Establishing the important factors—the first …**
That's right. The next is to be *comfortable*— *comfortable* within yourself. That is important.	**And the second …**
The third is to be *confident*. You *know* that you can do this job, you are very *confident* of that.	**And the third**
So those are the three important things. Let's think about them one by one. (*Nods*)	

Staying *calm*. You have learned how to breathe easily, breathing away tightness and tension, so let yourself imagine that you are getting seated in the interview room, and you can focus on breathing easily and comfortably. That's right. Focus only on your breathing, for a few moments, until you feel settled. Let me know when that has happened. (*Nods*) That's very good. Can you feel that sense of calmness within yourself and your body? (*Nods*) I knew that you knew how to do that, and you see—you really do know. It's good to have that deep self-assurance, hmmm? And that adds to your sense of calmness.

Now pay a little more attention towards being really *comfortable* within your body and your mind. It is important to feel comfortable in *both* mind and body, isn't it? Yes. That's right.

And now for the third "C"—*confidence*. Go deep within yourself, to the very core of yourself, where all your strengths and talents are stored, and find that essence of *confidence*. Just let it pour right into your heart and mind, so strongly that you can actually *feel* it pouring in. (*Watch, and she perhaps smiles or settles down even more*)

So now you know that you have tapped into all three—*calmness*, *comfort* and *confidence*—the three vital "Cs" that offer the best possible interview, and the best chance for that job.

And you know that you can practice at home, to keep the Cs strong within you, and you can always enjoy the support of the other parts of you, too, that want to help you. You know who those helping parts are, and you can look forward to accepting their support. Now just bring yourself out of hypnosis in your own way.

Re-establishing a well-known technique—the first "C"

Recognizing the sense of calmness—notice the self and the body, which strengthens the overall impression in more than one dimension

Onto the second "C"

Again, two aspects, "mind *and* body"—both are important

And the third "C", to be found "where all your strengths and talents are stored"—emphasizing that the client already has many strengths and this is simply one more which can be accessed

Reiterating the message

Every practice helps the end result to be very positive

Carefully enlisting the support of **other ego states, who may have been feeling left out**

Getting along together—inside

As therapy progresses, so does the opportunity for some ego states to feel left out or less important than how they perceive the other ego states to be. There is often considerable vying for attention as the weeks go by, and what had seemed to be a tight-knit inner community may seem to be fraying a bit at the seams.

Some therapists perceive this as a good thing—a chance to begin resolution and/or integration. Personally, I disagree, as it seems to me to be more of a "growing up" situation, not unlike adolescent sibling rivalry. Viewed in that perspective, we can think of it as a stage of the maturing process, *after which* resolution or integrative techniques have a better chance of taking root.

There has seemed to be a bit of anxiety between all of Mary's parts, lately. Does that also seem how it is to you? (*Nods of agreement, perhaps reluctantly*)	**Recognizing the situation and bringing it up in a matter-of-fact way**
Would you like to find a better way to work together, as you have been doing lately over other issues? (*Nods of agreement—again, perhaps with some reluctance*)	**Making sure that you and the client (and her ego states) are on the same track**
Alright. How about this: those of you who would like to find a better way to work together can do so, and the others can, for now, just watch. How does that sound? (*More nods, with more assurance*)	**Allowing independence between the ego states. This also encourages trust that you are not on one side or the other**
Fine. So, some of you can think of one or two situations where you are not in the same ballpark, and you agree that some way to work together would be better. Is that right? (*Nods*)	**Opening the door to negotiation**
Then that is a very workable situation. Can you let me know how many of you are feeling that way? (*Some sort of signal or comment is made*)	**Acknowledging their willingness to work together, and asking for some information regarding an important factor**

Three of you. That is an excellent start. Now you can talk about it out loud, so that I can hear you, or just within yourself, whatever seems most safe for you. Nod if you wish to do this privately. (*Nods*)

Reassurance.
Offering the chance to do it privately if they feel strongly about that. It could be perceived as dangerous to "tell" out loud

I am going to presume that they are going to do this silently. If they are willing to do it out loud, then a different approach is used, which I shall describe later.

Then I shall be quiet for a little while—just a few minutes by clock time, but as long as you need in hypnosis time. I'll keep track of the clock time for you. Is that alright with you? (*Nods*) Good.

This ploy works very well, as time is very often misperceived in hypnosis anyway, according to what the subject needs, and/or his or her emotional involvement in the situation

I usually allow about three or four minutes for these changes to come together. More than that and the client will probably be drifting off on a different tangent. Throughout that few minutes I make the appropriate comments: "About half of the clock time is over now ... About three-quarters of the clock time is over now ..." etc.

Now stay in hypnosis, but come back into present time. That's right.

It is important to make sure that this has happened

Before we close the hypnosis for now, you may want to decide on some small situation where you can find out how this new way of working together actually works. That can be exciting, so look forward to it, and maybe you'll have something to tell me the next time we meet, here in my office.

There's nothing better than actually getting started! So give a positive post-hypnotic suggestion that will encourage that to happen

And the suggestion that she will tell you!

If the client decides that she wants to keep you informed as the session goes on, so that the communication between the ego states is out loud, making the comments vague seems to work best: "Mmm", "Um-hum", "Ahhh", with just enough emphasis to reassure the client that you are attending to the process and agreeing with it. If you do not agree with it, gently intervene with a mild suggestion: "Yes, that would be one way to approach it. Can you think of an alternative, too?"

At times the conversation between the parts can become quite vigorous, so be prepared with some neutralizing ploys that you can call on if necessary: "These are interesting things that you are discussing. Maybe you could even take a moment or two to think about how it would work in a real situation. Then you'll be even better prepared."

Blending

Blending is the term I use that refers to the *temporary* joining of two or more ego states in order to achieve a special task or function. The important word to remember is "temporary". The ego states themselves have the jurisdiction to undo the blend at any time.

This serves several uses: for example, it offers a means by which one ego state, who knows how to do something, can teach another ego state who needs to know how to do that same something, a format in which that can happen. It also offers an opportunity for the client to find out what it's like for their ego states to work together so closely that they are working as "one"—in other words, a rehearsal for integration, if the client decides to go down that route, or (more likely) resolution.

For every dissociative client with whom I have worked, being offered this gift—of the power to choose—has meant a great deal. It also establishes a good rapport between therapist and client, and improves the level of trust. It is not appropriate, however, until one is well into the second stage of therapy and most, if not all, of the personality structure is known by both therapist and client.

Settle yourself comfortably in the chair and take yourself into hypnosis in your own way. You know how to do that.	**Getting settled in the usual, familiar way**
Let yourself reach that level in which you can learn how to do something new, that could be very useful for you.	**Setting the scene for some new and important technique**
We know that (Mary) and (Phyllis) often work together, and that together they can achieve great results. Perhaps there is a way that they can do that even more effectively. I call it *blending,* and you remember I spoke about it (last week).	**It is always the client who chooses the ingredients of the blend, although the therapist can make suggestions**
Do you both now feel that you would like to learn how to do that? (*They nod*)	**Making sure that they are ready to explore this possibility (which may seem very strange to them)**

Good.

You remember that you yourselves are in control of the blending, and that you can dissolve it whenever you choose to do so. Is that right? (*Signals "yes"*)

Good.

Now, I don't know exactly how you are going to achieve the blend, because everybody does it a little bit differently. You may want to explore a few possibilities now, in your hypnosis. Would that be helpful? We discussed them before, but it's always a little different to hear about it in hypnosis.

For example, you may feel that you can just merge into each other for a short, temporary period of time. See how that might work for you. I'll be quiet while you explore that, and then become your separate selves again. Nod or lift a finger when you are finished

(*When you have received the message*)
Um-hum

Would you like another possibility?

Alright. Sometimes, it can be more like feeling close to each other when you seem really connected. Find out how that feels, and then become your separate selves again, and nod or lift a finger when you are finished.

(*When you have received the message*)
Um-hum.

Would you like to explore one more possibility? (*Yes*)

Reinforcing that this is *their* choice

Again, it is personal and their choice

Hypnosis is the ideal way to explore

Offering possibilities. Be prepared to offer several

Ideomotor responses are very useful and are less interruptive than speaking

Of course, we each have our own suggestions. These are just some examples

Alright. In your own way, make bonds between you, so snug that they are nice and comfortable, and very secure. Then, when you are ready, become your separate selves again, and let me know by nodding or lifting a finger.

Three possibilities seem to be a useful number

(*When you have received the message*)
Very good.

Now, you have explored three different ways in which you could blend together, *temporarily,* in order that you can learn how to do something even better than you could do it before. So choose now which of the three feels best for you, and blend together in the way which feels just right. Nod or lift a finger to let me know that you have achieved that blend.

Reinforcing that it is her choice, not yours, and that it is *temporary,* and under her control

(*When you have received the message*)
Very good. Stay together, blended for just a little while. I'm going to let you know when one full minute has passed. Is that alright? (*Wait for the response*)

Rehearsal for staying in the blended state, which they will have to do when they are doing this themselves

Very good indeed. Now, just take another minute and make sure that that way of blending feels comfortable. Let me know.

Reinforcing their control

FIRST POSSIBLE RESPONSE: POSITIVE

How well you have learned that! Just practice here in my office one more time. Do your blend, let me know when you have achieved that, and I'll advise you one full minute later.

Good for you! An achievement!

One full minute seems to be a good length of time—not too long but long enough

Very good indeed.

Now, you can practice this at home, as long as it feels comfortable doing that. Remember, the choice is yours. If you decide to practice at home, stay in your blend for a little while and then unblend. Does that feel alright for you?

It is important to practice but they may not feel quite comfortable about doing this on their own just yet

(*Nod or finger response*) Very good indeed.

SECOND POSSIBLE RESPONSE: NEGATIVE

Now, that's very good. You have realized that you are not quite ready to do that yet, or that we haven't found exactly the right pathway to blending for you. Because soon it will be time for us to finish this session today, take the whole idea home and think it over. Perhaps you yourself might know a much better way to do the blending—if you *want* to do some blending. We can talk about it next time

Emphasizing that you respect their sense of what is right for them

(*Then invite the client to come out of hypnosis in their own way.*)

Getting along together—outside

It is one thing for the ego states to learn how to get along together on the inside, but it is another to learn how to get along together on the outside. It requires a level of social comfort, knowing that other people are watching and observing, that is quite different from the internal organization.

First script

Carla and Carly, you've been telling me— if I'm right about the interpretation—that you would like to sample what it's like to "get along together" on the *outside*, that is, in the real world, where outside people are watching and interpreting your behaviour. Are you still interested in exploring it at this time? (*Signals yes*)

Making sure that you're on the same wavelength, and that she hasn't changed her mind

Differentiating "inside" collaboration from "outside" collaboration

Alright. Then let's do a little experiment. First of all, the two of you blend, as you know how to do. Let me know when you have achieved that blend. (*Nods*) Good.

Starting with something she knows how to do

Now, *stay blended*, and open your eyes and come out of hypnosis in your own way, but *still blended*, and find out how that feels.

Now for the variation on the theme—quite a different situation

("*It feels very strange,*" *the blended pair respond,* "*but it's okay, just very strange. I just didn't realize it would feel so strange—as if we're just one person—it's peculiar.*")

Normalizing a strange effect

Yes, I'm sure it does feel peculiar. Did you realize that you just spoke of the blended pair of you as "I"? (*Look of bewilderment on the client's face*) Um-hum. I'm not surprised that that surprised you! But you did. So you have accomplished something very new today: staying blended on the *outside*, which is really a brand new awareness. And that brief interlude is all we need to do today. We can practice again in a few days, or even tomorrow, if you wish to do so.

Supporting her response and also pointing out *another* peculiarity

Usually it is better to do this in several small episodes, so as not to overwhelm her

Now, go back inside, *still blended*, and find your level of blended comfort. That's right, very good. Stay in the blend for a little longer, and then unblend if you wish to do so, or just stay blended until you choose to unblend, back on the inside.

Back into familiar territory—so she can relax and stay blended at the same time

Remember that blending is always a *temporary* choice, to achieve some particular purpose. You've done very well today—you are literally learning how to get along in a new way, *outside*.

Blending is always temporary, the length of time being the choice of the client, *not* the therapist

Second script

Carla and Carly, you have been doing well, practicing that whole new way of getting along together on the outside, by blending first, and then coming out of your hypnosis while still blended. It has been an interesting experience for you, and a new skill that you now know that you have. And I think that it is also a little bit of fun—am I right? (*Signals yes*)

It is important to make sure that she has been practicing; if you have reason to doubt it, repeat the first exercise (presuming that she wants to do that). Most often, it has been a little bit of excitement in a controlled and safe environment

Well, that's very nice. Now you are ready
to practice the next step, and that means
interacting with other people who are on
the outside while you are in a blend. Do
you feel ready to explore that new skill?

**This is a delicate question—she
wants to, but it is a bit scary**

(Obviously some consideration going on, then a Yes signal.)

Alright. We'll make it easy for you and
you can start by interacting with me as the
outside person. This will be easier as you
already know me. (*Probably she will show
some lessening of tension*)

**She knows you and feels safe
with you, so it is a good way to
start**

So go into your blend, as you know how
to do, and let me know when you are
comfortably there. Yes? Good.

**She knows how to do this
herself by this time. If she
doesn't, go back a step**

Now, *stay blended*, and come out of your
hypnosis in your own blended way. Good.
Here you are. Talk to me in your blended
state, and tell me how it feels.

**Encourage her to come out of
hypnosis a little more slowly
than usual**

*You can now have a short—three or four minutes—conversation during which
the blended pair can converse with you. You'll have to do the leading, probably,
asking general questions that will not challenge them too much. However, there
are always exceptions, and this blended pair might be very happy indeed to be
having a conversation with you, as "she" explores a new state of being. Use your
intuition and be ready to close the conversation when you sense that it is time to
do so. Then invite the blended pair to go back into hypnosis, unblend if they choose
to do so, and then come out of hypnosis in their own way.*

*Usually, if the blend fits well, they will choose to stay blended, often for quite a
long time, and getting along well on both the inside and outside, until they are
ready to consider resolution or even integration. At other times, they will blend
just to cope with a specific situation, and when that is resolved they will separate
again.*

More about blending

At times, a client may wish to have a "temporarily permanent" blend,
rather than having to do it over and over again, as sometimes happens.

One of my clients was in such a situation, and she has given me permission (anonymously) to use this very nice procedure which she thought of herself. I have simply adapted it into the third person, instead of the first person. The explanations are the way she described it to me. When she first came into my practice, she had many ego states and for many years she was very unwilling to give any of them up, as they each filled an important role for her. But this way, she explained, they learned to get along together and found that they could achieve more that way than when they stayed separate.

But it is still up to her to decide if and when they will permanently merge. I feel that this is the way blending evolved into resolution for her. There are still three powerful ego states that have not entered the blend, and they fill very functionary roles within her system.

Think of a river. It comes from far away, the top of a mountain, and starts with a little stream, maybe from snow melting or something like that.	**Setting the scene, evolving the metaphor**
As it travels down the mountain, other little streams join it, so that by the time it gets down the mountain to the valley below, it is quite a bit bigger than when it started out. Most of the little streams joining in are quite small, but some of them are deeper, wider, stronger, as if they have an important purpose.	**Some of the ego states join the river, adding to its strength, width and depth** **This is an important statement. When joined, they can achieve more than when separate**
Some of them even have a bit of an undertow, and they add that undertow to the much larger river that now courses through the valley.	**An added quality**
From time to time, a little rivulet drifts from the large river for some reason—because it meets a little road block, like a rock that the river has to go around. Sometimes, when a little river separates, it rejoins the river later, but sometimes not, at least not right away. Perhaps it runs alongside the big river, or goes in its own direction. Maybe it wasn't ready to join the big river, yet.	**It is too soon, perhaps, for some of the ego states to be comfortable in the blended state** **It may "run alongside" in order to discover more about the big river. Big rivers can be dangerous**

It's hard to know where or when this river will eventually meet the ocean, but for now it is enough that it is there, strong and purposeful.

No one knows how long this blend will last, but for now, it is useful

It is a good river.

Validation of the concept

The Maypole Blend
(Only for those who are old enough to know what a maypole is!)

This is a simple little procedure for clients who want to toy with the idea of a blend. They are perhaps intrigued with the idea, but not quite sure about it. It could be an idea to offer those who gave a negative response as to whether they were ready to stay with the blending or stay separate all the time. Because it is quite short, it can be offered when the appointment time is not quite up. It is done with the client already in hypnosis *or* simply sitting in the chair, imagining the situation with their eyes closed.

(Caution: some clients have been subjected to rituals, and the maypole dance could possibly be reminiscent. It's a stretch, but think about it.)

Think of a maypole, with many dancers each finding a ribbon to grasp. There are many different colours of ribbons. When each participant is holding the end of a ribbon, the dance begins.

Describing the scene

The ego states who wish to participate in the dance grasp a ribbon

First, everybody just dances, circling around the maypole, holding the ribbon, all going in the same direction

The therapist may wish to put a lilt in their voice

After a little time, half the dancers turn to face the opposite way, and then the dancers start to weave in and out, so the ribbons become entwined. It forms a pretty pattern down the pole, with the colours going in and out.

There is more than one way to do this dance (maybe more ego states wish to participate)

Sometimes the dancers want to make it even more complex, so that perhaps a third of the dancers face one way and two thirds another way. There are many possible patterns to the dance.

Many ego states join the dance around the maypole

But in time, the music is coming to a close and it is time to undo the weave, simply by going backwards to the beginning. And then the maypole is plain again and the ribbons hang gently, waiting for the next dance.

The dance (the blend) is temporary. It is easy to undo

Integration or resolution?

As people approach the end of their therapeutic journey, there is always the question: Do you want integration or resolution?

Neither of these eventualities can happen until the following criteria have been achieved:

* All amnesia barriers are down
* Everybody knows everybody else in the system
* There are no more secrets in the system
* There is no more internal sabotage or self-harm
* All major decisions are made by the adults in the system
* All children (child parts) are protected

Integration: all the various ego states begin to link up so that they are working as one functional unit—much like the usual understanding or ordinary ego states in non-dissociative people.

Resolution: the ego states continue to function independently, but in cooperation with all the other ego states, adhering to the criteria above.

Generally, if the system chooses resolution, no specific hypnotic techniques are necessary. However, a simple encouraging hypnosis may be helpful.

Preparing for resolution

If this is the first time you have decided to use hypnosis to specifically address the beginnings of resolution—i.e. getting along together inside— then some introduction to the idea must first have been made and agreement reached that the client is ready to consider this part of the healing process. There is often considerable reluctance on the part(s) of some of the ego states, so great care must be taken to assure both yourself and the client, that this is now a good time to begin, and that the client is ready to do this. The concept of resolution is a tricky business because although the client will be relieved to know that the therapist is not going to insist on *integration*—a concept that many clients will regard in a negative light—the very idea of any kind of merging can be scary. This is even more frightening if the client perceives, rightly or wrongly, that the therapist is going to use hypnosis to trick them into something about which they are not fully comfortable.

Susan, we've talked about the use of hypnosis to explore the idea of resolution. Do you, yourself, feel ready to begin that exploration? Signal to me if that is alright with you.	**Reminding her that you have discussed this before, and remembering that it may have been a different ego state(s) with whom you had the earlier discussion**
(*Presuming you get a positive signal*) Good. Then, let's begin.	
You may wish to go a little further into hypnosis, or even perhaps come back to a lighter level. Just make sure that you are at a comfortable level. (*Nods*)	**Settling into a level of hypnosis that is comfortable for everyone is very important; although there may be two main players, others are listening, too**
So settle yourself into that comfortable place in your hypnosis, and find the two parts of you that are interested and wish to explore this possibility. Let me know when you feel ready. (*Nods*)	**It works best when they choose the main players themselves**
Next, choose a situation on which you both believe that you can agree. Then, when you have done that, discuss the situation with each other, and discover whether there are some aspects that need a little more thought before you are both comfortable. You can do this silently or aloud. Remember, it is quite alright for you to each have your own ideas.	**It is important that the ego states agree on this choice**
	Checking for mutual agreement
	Reinforcing the concept that one or the other might have a different perspective, and that is fine and, often, useful

What is needed is an agreement that you can agree to work together. There are times when it is useful for a different perspective to be brought forth and then discussed, so that a mutually agreeable decision or solution can be found. However you choose to do it, let me know when you have reached a comfortable decision. (*A time lapse, then a nod or other signal*)

Working on the solution or situation

That is excellent—a good piece of work. Come out of your hypnosis in your own way now so that we can talk about your experiences.

This is long enough for a first time—a good introduction to the idea, which they can now discuss

More about preparation for resolution

As I have stated previously, by the time the client is preparing for resolution, they will probably already be acquainted with the process of blending. If not, blending is an important asset when working towards resolution and the therapist may want to consider helping them to achieve these talents. For some reason, I have found that women clients are more likely to choose these skills than men.

Well, Susan, you have come a long way during the time we've been working together, and you have decided to explore the possibility of resolution. Do you still feel that way? (*Yes*)

Pointing out her achievements, and making sure that she is ready for this next, very important step

I think that it's a good idea, too. Do you feel comfortable about using hypnosis as an aid to achieving that goal? (*Yes*) Alright. Then go into hypnosis now, as you know how to do, and let me know when you feel that you are at a comfortable level. (*Wait for the signal*) Good. Do a little relaxation first, just so that you feel settled. Remember that we are just exploring today—discovering whether it might be suitable for you.

Again, assuring her comfort level; she can do this herself
A little relaxation always helps

More reassurance that this is just exploring, not written in stone

Now, this experience today is for the adults—everybody who is over 19 years of age. So make sure, before we go any further, that all the children are comfortable, safe, and are being cared for. Let me know when you know that that has happened. Good.

Clarifying the boundaries

Very important to make sure that child ego states are in a safe place

Each of you knows that you all have talents and experiences that are special for you. And you have already had many experiences where someone has had to make a decision. That will also be the case when you all work towards resolution. So just think about that, for a minute or so by clock time—take as long as you like in your hypnosis time—and then give further thought as to whether a Board of Directors you suit you better or a kind of communal coming-to-an-agreement arrangement suits your needs. Either can work very well as long as everybody is comfortable with whatever the decision is. (*After a short interval*) It seems as if you have arrived at a decision. Can you tell me what the decision is?

The concept of decision-making may or may not have come up— at least, not so specifically—so do it now

Hypnosis time and clock time may be far away from each other

Decisions about decisions—very important at this stage

You may think that you already know, but she might surprise you, so make sure of her choice

(*After you have understood the decision*) That sounds as if it will work very well for you. Let's rehearse, then, and see what is feels like when you put that decision into practice. To do that, you can either come out of hypnosis or go into an eyes-open hypnosis. You can choose what feels best for you at this time. Remember, you are *rehearsing*, rather than writing something in stone.

Either way, she is preparing for a new level of awareness, and of working as a unit within the whole personality structure

At this stage, there are two possible scenarios, and either can be done with eyes-open hypnosis or out of hypnosis, but each involves the whole system.

BOARD OF DIRECTORS DECISION

You have decided, together, on having a Board of Directors. So let's do an imaginary scenario and see how it works. Is that alright with you? (*Yes*)

Getting started, by exploring some possible scenarios

First, have you decided on the Chair of the Board? If not, then that is your first decision. Are you going to do it by an election or a consensus? (*Somebody may say, "We think Jane should be the Chair—she understands this stuff."*)

Very often, the ego states have *not* chosen a Chair, and it is crucial to do so as soon as possible. You are offering options, but not too many: the comment is just as likely to be "we need an election"

Good. So that possibility should work well, then. Now, let's look a different kind of situation: Mary believes that she has the possibility of a job. This means the whole group will have to re-organize around that decision, so it's a good idea to get the go-ahead from the Board before she signs on. Does that sound as if it would be a good example? (*Yes*)

The client, and her parts, may not have thought this through, so point it out right from the beginning, giving some examples of how it might evolve

Then discuss some situation that might come up if she does accept the job. What might that be? (*We'll all have to get up at the same time!*) Yes, that's a good thought to begin with. Now, you folks on the Board discuss this, aloud or not as you choose, and come to a decision. Then let me know.

It is useful to watch the facial expressions, to get an idea of how things are going

Simple scenarios such as these (which may not be so simple!) can be suggested by the therapist as try-out situations. Make sure suggestions are realistic, taking the client's personality structure, capabilities and endurance into consideration.

CONSENSUS DECISION

A consensus can be a wonderful way to get everybody working together, so let's see how it could work out. Choose a situation in which a decision is needed, then find out whether the consensus worked for you. Do you have some suggestions?

Validating the decision

The first decision!—to choose a situation. Is it done by vote or by consensus?

Presuming a decision has been made and accepted:

Now, I'll keep quiet while you come to
your consensus; let me know when have
done that.

*If the client cannot decide on a typical situation, you may ask, after some time
during which a choice could have been made, whether you could offer a suggestion,
just to get the process started. If the answer is "yes", then an idea similar to the one
above could be used. Either way, tell the client that they have done very well in this
early exploration.*

So you have begun to understand what
consensus means, and how you can use
it as you begin working together. It is a
new challenge—but you have faced many
challenges before, and this is just the
beginning of the next step in your healing
journey.

**Validation of the work done and
reassurance for the future**

A different situation

This is another prelude towards resolution.

As the various ego states learn how to get along together inside, some
degree of mutual satisfaction begins to emerge. When this begins to
happen more possibilities for working together come to the forefront. One
of these is for *more than two* ego states to work together on some project.
As always, this readiness must come from within the system, not from the
outside.

You will appreciate that this is quite different from blending, which is
temporary joining of two or more ego states for some specific purpose.
This script is for those clients who are close to deciding on resolution
rather that integration. The ego states retain their individuality but work
together.

The script may be used in hypnosis, or not, as the client chooses.

Anna, you and Annette and Annie seem to be interested in working together on the writing project. It seems, at least to me, as if the three of you are offering suggestions. Am I correct in this interpretation? (*Some sign or comment indicating that this is the correct interpretation*)

Identifying the possibilities of some mutual interaction—and checking it out

Um-hum. What is it that intrigues you all? Can you tell me?

Asking for more information in order to be able to help

(*Some response from the client, offering a suggestion or two as to how they might work together—this must come from inside.*)

Ah, I see. Yes, that seems like a good idea as it does involve the three of you. Do you have as plan as to how to begin?

Often, good ideas collapse when there is no starting point

Hmmm. How about taking a little time out to discuss a possible starting point. (*Nods*) Do you want to do that in your hypnosis or out of hypnosis?

Do it whichever away they want—it is *their* project

(*Either having stayed in hypnosis or now back in hypnosis.*)

Now, the three of you can take a little time and plan how you are going to begin. The beginning of a project is obviously a very important step. Take your time and share your views. Remember, everybody's views are equally important, and you can choose, together, those that seem to offer a workable starting point. I'm going to keep quiet for a little while, to give you time to do this. Just let me know when you are ready to tell me something.

Initiating the planning stage

Sharing **is the important word here, as it is like a brainstorming session in that anything goes and great ideas can evolve from very simple suggestions (this is one of my favorite techniques)**

(*The client indicates that the three ego states have come to some decision. This might take two minutes or fifteen—in the latter case, you might suggest that they could "push the pause button", as they can do when, for example, something needs to be put on hold in the middle of a meeting or when they are involved in some detailed work and have to leave it temporarily unfinished.*)

Our session is running out of time. Would you prefer to carry on with this yourselves until our next session? Or would you rather keep the pause button engaged?

This statement serves the dual purpose of keeping to limits and of offering choices as to how to do that

Further preparation for resolution

Jeanette, just settle yourself down and let everybody get comfortable. Go into hypnosis as far as you wish at this time, and do a little breathing exercise to help the hypnosis process.

Giving time to get settled

That's right.

Now you have all reached the stage where you know each other and are comfortable with each other. You've shared your histories and given each other support. From now on—and it has already begun— all the grown-ups in the system will be functioning like a well-organized Board of Directors, discussing what is best for everybody for the situations that come up from day to day.

Reaffirming that this is something the system already knows how to do—emphasizing the concept of supporting each other
Reminding them that this is for the adults in the system

When situations come up that may cause some disagreement between you, for example, as to how it might best be handled, then you can discuss it very respectfully together and reach a clear, satisfactory conclusion that everybody can feel comfortable with.

Again emphasizing the *respectful* aspect—very important

Just take a few moments, now, to think back over the past few weeks, and think of the times when you were all doing this spontaneously. I'll be quiet for a few moments, while you do that.

Relating this to what she/they already know

(*After ten seconds or so*) That's right. So you can understand the concept, as you know that you can do, because you have been doing it now for quite a while anyway, without even knowing it or putting a name to it. And that's wonderful!—does everybody agree? You already know how to do what you need to know how to do.

Hypno-speak again—and it works!

You can take a little time, maybe later on today or maybe tomorrow, to think of this again, and then it can become part of your combined strength, that you can all do together for the benefit of everybody.

Preparing for integration

It will be important to speak with the whole system first (*"Now, everybody listen!"*) and confirm that this is what they all—even the child parts—want to do. A child part that does *not* want to integrate can sabotage the whole process.

Settle yourselves comfortably into the chair and take yourselves into hypnosis—all together—in your own way. Be sure that *everybody* goes into hypnosis.

This is important because at times an unhappy part will (silently) refuse to join

When you are all in hypnosis, ask each other whether you want to integrate into one person, while keeping your own particular gifts and contributions, because each of you *do* bring your own gifts, your own strengths and ideas to the system.

"Keeping your own gifts ..." is crucial reassurance

That's right. You can understand how important it is to recognize your own contribution, and those of all the others, also. Everybody's contribution is very, very important.

More crucial reassurance

Now perceive an image of yourselves beginning to merge into a single entity, in the most pleasant, comfortable way. People do this in many ways, so your way is very personal to you.

It doesn't matter what the image is, as long as there *is* an image

Take your time. Remember, you are all, each part, a very, very important part of the whole being.

Ego strengthening of the whole new ego structure

Let me know when you perceive, at a deep, subconscious way, that you have merged.

Merging may happen fairly quickly or much more slowly. If it is taking a very long time, you can suggest that the subconscious is wisely taking time to explore what it is going to feel like, and maybe that is all that needs to be done today. If that is the case, invite them to go back into their separate selves again and, in a few minutes, re-alert them from their hypnosis. After the return to the here and now, discuss how long the wait should be before exploring the union concept again.

When merging has occurred:

You have done a splendid job. Now it is time to come gently out of your hypnosis and find out how it feels to be a unity— one person, with many facets to our own personality but all together as one person.

"Gently" is the important word

Be prepared for any of several possibilities: a dissolving of the union, a need to have it strengthened, an internal war, a perceived change in the way they present to the world, happiness, sort-of-happiness, distress or many other possibilities.

Another way to achieve integration is to have several similar parts merge, over a period of time, until there are three of our larger "parts" of the ego structure. Then, in time, these can merge into one. Often, for example, child parts can merge easily and become one or two "large" child parts.

Your client will probably need to keep in close touch with you for several weeks after integration. The world will seem a very strange place to them. As one presenter at a meeting several years ago described it—"I have never lived in this world before."

Section IV

Children

Almost all children go into hypnosis in the blink of an eye, as they live in their imaginations much of the time anyway.

This is both a blessing and a curse, because going into an altered state of consciousness is also what they do to get away from the abuse. It is particularly important, therefore, to watch for signals that they are in jeopardy of doing that while in hypnosis.

We always need to fit the hypnotic metaphor into the age and experience of the child. And is it also crucial to make sure that the child is no longer in the abusive home or situation. By the time they get into therapy, the child has almost always been removed from the traumatic surroundings, but it is still important to ascertain that this is the case.

It is also important to remember that many children—in fact, most—are very physically active during hypnosis. They shuffle around, pick their noses, open their eyes and look at the room and its furnishings, and all the time are still in hypnosis. It takes a little getting used to, but that's the way it often is. You can suggest, gently, that they close their eyes again, but they may or may not do that.

Important! The first part of this section is *not* about working with child ego states, but about working with children who come from abusive homes, and are usually, at this time, in the care of social services or foster parents. The child must be physically separated from their family in order for psychotherapy to help. Later scripts are about *teens who are dissociative*, not about teen ego states in an adult who has a dissociative disorder.

Most children are very upset about being separated from their families even though they have been, and probably were still being, abused in that environment. The abuse is "normal" for them. It's a sad world. It is not unusual for them to avoid going into a "formal" hypnosis at all, but choose to play with the Lego and create masterpieces of ingenuity. However, under all of that, they are listening; so just assume that they are in an altered state of consciousness (which they are) and proceed as if they were sitting calmly and politely on the "hypnosis" chair.

A new home for Jimmy

Jimmy, age 8, has recently been taken from his parental home and is with foster parents. He is angry and confused, and doesn't want to talk to anybody.

Jimmy, it's hard to have to move to a different house. Sometimes, though, it has to be done—and that's the case for you right now.	He is determinedly *not* listening; you keep on talking quietly
When that happens, and we are angry and upset, it's hard to figure out why it is happening and what it going to happen from now on.	The "we" is deliberate—it makes him feel that maybe he really is like some other people, after all
Sometimes, all we can do about it is start remembering the good times—when you were climbing the tree or playing with your dog. You can pretend that you are climbing again, but it is a different tree and so it is something new for you. And new things *can* be good things; we can all learn from new things.	Use whatever "good things" you might know about—the baseball team, going to the beach or some incident that was happy for him A positive suggestion
We'll probably be seeing each other a few more times, so you can think of things that you would like to talk about when you are here.	Preparing him for future visits *He* gets a chance to say what he wants to talk about

A script like this is very useful when a young child is using the play sandbox. Below is a script in which the sandbox is in his imagination.

A sandbox for Billy

Billy, do you remember, the last time that you were here, we talked about going into your imagination? (*Signals Yes*) I thought that we might do that for a few minutes today, and you can find out if you like it. Would that be okay? (*Signals Yes*)	Bringing the child into the process of decision-making

Good. So you can settle down into that very comfortable chair, and put your feet up, and close your eyes.

And in your imagination, maybe you can find a sandbox. (*Nods*) Let me know when you find it. (*Signals Yes*)

Most children respond to the suggestion

That's good—you found the sandbox very quickly. Maybe it was there hiding in your imagination all the time and all you had to do was tell yourself to find it! Do you think that that's what happened? (*May agree or disagree, or just shrug—let it go*)

Reinforcing his ability to do things himself

Well, anyhow, you found it! Now you can decide how you're going to ask the sandbox to help you to always feel safe and strong. Maybe there's an army in the sandbox, just waiting to help you; or maybe there's a very special dog to protect you. Or maybe there's something else that you may know about and I don't. If that's what is happening, can you tell me how the sandbox is going to help you feel safe? (*Signals Yes*)

He **makes the decision as to how he might do that**

Reinforcing that the sandbox *is* **helping and planting the seed in his imagination**

At this point, he may choose to tell you all about it, or not. You can question gently if you wish, but usually it's best to follow his lead. If he decides not to say anything, then just confirm that by saying that he can always tell you later, if he wants to. Many children enjoy keeping secrets from adults, and this is particularly the case with a child who—although he doesn't have the words to express it—feels that his whole mind is controlled by somebody else.

That's really just fine. Do you know that you can go and visit the sandbox anytime you want to, or need to? Especially if, for some reason, you want to feel safe? (*No*) Well, you can, because that sandbox is your own, special sandbox. It belongs to you, and nobody else. Isn't that a good thing to know? (*Signals Yes*)

Making sure that he knows that this is his own thing to do, and he doesn't have to wait for permission

I think so, too. And now it's time to come out of your nice daydream and back into my office, when I count to three. Alright? (*Signals Yes*) Good. One, two, three. Open your eyes and see where you are!

Re-alerting. Most children like a process (counting), rather than bringing themselves out in their own time

Rocket ship metaphor

This metaphor is usually better for boys than girls, although it can certainly be adapted if the young lady is particularly self-confident! It seems to work best for 8 to 12 year olds, but we all know that some children are older—or younger—that they seem. This is particularly true if he has been abused and has had to find ways to believe in himself and keep himself safe.

Jack, you've told me that sometimes you feel as if your whole life is controlled by other people; is that right? (*Yes*) So I'm going to describe a journey that you can go on by yourself, or take people that you know you want to take with you. Is that okay with you? (*Yes*)	**Both of you acknowledging the situation** **Giving him choices—very important**
Then, you'll be happy to know that this journey is on a spaceship. Yes! (*Almost all young boys brighten up at that remark!*) And I've never been on a spaceship, so you're going to have to make sure that I've said it right, or that you're able to change something if I've made a mistake. Okay? (*Yes—usually enthusiastically*)	**He will know that you've never been on a space ship, so he's the one making decisions here**
Alright. Then, in your own way, find your way to the spaceship and get aboard. Let me know when you're safely aboard. (*Signals*)	
Good. I think that you are going to be an officer on the ship—maybe you are even the Captain. Is that right? (*Yes*) Very good. So you into the Captain's chair and prepare for take off. Have you decided on your destination yet? Or are you going to wait and see how things are, out in space, and then decide? (*Usually he will answer*)	**Of course, he's the Captain—or Commanding Office or whatever category of rank best fits him** **He's in charge, he makes the choices**
Now, you can tell me what's happening, or you can keep it secret, but it's easier if I can understand what's happening. Is that okay? (*Yes*) Good. So you're taking off, starting your journey. And you are the one in control of that spaceship!	**Reinforcing that he is in control**

From here on, it will depend on where his imagination takes him. Probably there will be a bad guy that he has to subdue, or an insubordinate officer or crew member, or he needs to go far, far away from Earth because Earth is where the bad guys live. Male therapists may be better at this that female therapists—but we'll get our own back later.

This has been a very dramatic journey. But it's time now to come back to Earth, so do whatever you need to do to change your course and be homeward bound. Let me know when Earth is in sight. (*After a time, signals*)

Again, he is in charge

Good. Now bring your craft to a safe landing. It's been a good flight, hasn't it? (*Signals Yes*) And you are a very good Commanding Officer.

"Safe landing" is very important

Bolstering his capacity to make his own decisions (at least, sometimes)

You know, you can always go out on your spaceship again, because it belongs to you. Nobody else has the keys to open the door or get it started. So any time you need to go away for a while, you can have your spacecraft right there in your mind. Just do what we did here, settle down in a safe place, and take yourself on another journey. Because you know how to do that, now.

His ship, his choice

A suggestion that he *can* get away when things are too miserable

"You know how to do that, now"

I must give credit (and apologetic thanks) to Dr. Richard Kluft, who described a similar script at a meeting many years ago.

Promised not to tell

Many abused children are frightened into promising not to tell anybody what has happened or is happening to them. They are threatened that if they tell, terrible things will happen to them, or to their mothers, or to other people who are important to them, such as a favourite teacher. As the child has no way to assess this cognitively, they believe the abuser and do not tell. Often they are led to believe that they are very bad, anyway, and don't even deserve to have somebody to love them or care for them—just the abuser.

There is a way to get around such imperatives. Of course, it doesn't always work, but often it does so it's worth exploring.

The child is already in hypnosis—maybe with eyes open, maybe with eyes closed.

So Danny, you know that you have been told never to tell anybody about some of the things that grownup people are doing. (*Nods, often vigorously*) So I don't want you to tell me, either. But there's something that you *can* do instead. In fact, there are two or three things that you can do instead. I'm just going to tell you what they are, but you can decide whether you want to do them. Is that okay? (*Signals Yes—maybe warily*)

Establishing the situation
Offering some alternatives
(when he didn't know there were
any)

Here are some of the possibilities—Danny could:

- *whisper, not tell*
- *tell his dog or cat (he could have the animal with him in hypnosis)*
- *tell his favourite toy (he could be holding it, either really holding it or holding it in hypnosis)*
- *sing, not tell*
- *write it down, if he is old enough to do that*
- *draw a picture*
- *tell his favourite tree*
- *go into his tree house, in hypnosis, and tell his imaginary friend*

All of these possibilities are fraught with secrecy, which is the important element. Afterwards, you can say:

Danny, you are a very smart boy. You only told the cat, right? Good for you. You can even keep it secret from (*the abuser*) that you told (the cat), because the cat is a cat and so you kept your promise

Establishing the child-logic that
he can use

Now, maybe the cat will tell somebody—
that's up to the cat, whether he does that,
but you have kept the secret, as you were
told to do. And if (*the bad man/woman*)
asks you, you can honestly say that you
kept the secret from everybody else.

Answering the "but what if …"

So you can feel more comfortable now. Do
you want to come out of hypnosis? (*Yes*)
Alright, then come back into this room
and open your eyes.

Concluding the session

Hello! Nice to see you!

You were away! Now you're back!

I suggest that you avoid saying, "But you can tell me …", because you are "somebody" and it will place him in a potentially dangerous dilemma.

For the teenager

The teens face a difficult dilemma. They know that they aren't children any more, and feel that they have to pretend to be adults. If they have a highly dissociative ego system, they may well have a major role in that system. (It is common for dissociative clients to have ego states who are *older* than the client.) It is vital, therefore, to make very, very sure of what it is that they want to accomplish. To complicate things further, although they may be teens in reality, i.e. they were born twelve to eighteen years ago, in the system they may be an entirely different age. Clear discussion is imperative, being very respectful of their role, whatever that might be. If their goal is to be able to kill off the abuser, for instance, firmly refuse the opportunity!

Ben, we've talked about hypnosis and
you've said that you want to learn how
to do some of that. Do you still feel that
way? (*Yes*)

Clarifying his willingness

Okay. Then tell me what it is that you
would like to achieve, using hypnosis to
help you.

There's no point in focusing on something he doesn't want

Some possibilities to consider:

- *Feeling stronger*
- *Learning how to do something better than before*
- *Learning how to value his self-respect*
- *Understanding his own role better (e.g. he is responsible for his own safety, but not of his mother's or that of his siblings—this is often very difficult for him to accept)*
- *In general terms, how trauma affects someone's brain*

I'll use one of these as an example.

I know that you feel that you're responsible for keeping other people in your family safe. But the most important thing that you can do, for yourself and for them, is to keep *yourself* safe. You have to be safe yourself, if you want to help them. Is that right? (*Nods his head, perhaps reluctantly*)

He will feel that he is abandoning them, which is a terrible thought for him; he needs to counteract that impression—with your help

So, to keep yourself safe, you need to be *very* sure of what's going on around you. That will help you to help others in your family, too. Just think about that for a minute or so, while I keep quiet. Think about how to be *very* sure of what's going on around you.

The logical reasoning

(*After about a minute of silence*) That's good. Do you need a little more time? (*Nods or shakes head; proceed appropriately, giving another minute or carrying on*)

Have you thought about some good ways to keep yourself safe? (*Yes*)

Often these "ways" seem very nebulous; if you are talking about them afterwards, just nod your head as if they are the epitome of good reasoning

Good. Perhaps, after we finish the hypnosis, you can tell me about them, if you want to. Or, you can wait for a while and tell me when you're ready. It's your own decision, about when to tell me. Does that sound like a good idea? (*Signals Yes*) Good.

Important for him to feel that he makes his own decisions, but you have set the scene

I'll just keep quiet for another minute or so, in case there's something more that you'd like to spend a little more time on, then I'll invite you to come out of hypnosis.

I have purposely kept this vague, as it will be different for each client. It is just a skeleton to build on. He desperately needs to strengthen his self-image, partly because he feels responsible for what happens to others in the family, and partly to strengthen his own sense of self.

Sports

Sports metaphors are extremely useful and very appropriate to use in these situations. Do your best to know something about the sport you are describing! It helps if it is one of the sports that the youngster enjoys—either playing themselves or watching on TV. Of course, if you are not a sports geek, you can always turn it around and ask the young client to explain it to you. Personally, as a non-sports geek, I find that it works well.

Tanya, last week we were talking about the Olympic swimming finals. You were very interested in them. Do you like swimming, too? (*Yes*)

Setting the scene

It's a great sport for you. (*Nods*) Just close your eyes for a few minutes, so you can take yourself to one of those final races. You can pretend that you are one of the swimmers. Let me know when you really feel like you are there. (*Takes her time, then nods*)

Personal interaction

Is it a final race? (*No*) Ah. Then you have an even better chance of doing well, don't you? (*Nods*)

A way to make the waiting positive

Take your time, and find out how the race goes. I'm thinking that you'll do pretty well. Tell me when you're about to start the last lap. (*Nods*)

Positive suggestion

Good. And you're well prepared, too, because you've been practising. Tell me what's happening as you do your final lap.

More positive suggestion(s)

(*She begins to talk like a sportscaster, following it yard after yard after yard as she sprints for the finish line. <u>You</u> keep encouraging her, listening for the metaphor and responding to it. "That's it—you're nearly there, you can see the finish line and you know that you're going to win, that's right, nobody can keep you back now, you're getting closer and closer—there! It's just ahead of you—there! You've done it!"*)

You can feel what's it's like to overcome all the odds, is that right? That was a really splendid race. Have you ever noticed that sometimes it feels familiar, watching a race, or being in one? As if you've been there before, but not sure when that was? When that happens, it's often that deep, wise part of our minds that connects real life with our imaginations.

Overcoming odds is what she has been doing for a long time; this is a nice way to recognize it

Suggestion for conscious/ subconscious connection

I think that it's our subconscious, helping us to understand something that may be hard to understand. And maybe we begin to understand it before we even *know* that we've already understood it. Sometimes it takes a long time for us to realize something and then, one day, we *do* understand it. You may discover that yourself, some day.

Time distortion—a tried and true hypnotic technique

Implied suggestion, which works very well after time distortion

Obviously this basic script can be modified into any kind of sports activity.

Getting well

The therapeutic journey for children and teens is usually much shorter than it is for adults. But we can never presume that it will just happen without some specific effort on our part. Making a positive suggestion within a hypnotic session can help.

You know, Liz, we've been working together for quite a long time, and you've certainly worked hard. I think that you can be very proud of yourself, because you are so much clearer in your thinking and understanding, now. Is that true? (*Nods*)

Offering well-deserved kudos

Um-hum. So maybe it's a good time to start thinking about that. Do you have a kind of intuition, some kind of a feeling about when you'll be just fine working on your own, without me? (*May indicate Yes or No, or may not*) Or maybe just coming to see me every now and then if you want to? (*Nods Yes—this feels safer*)

Helping her set the scene

Implication that this will, indeed, happen

So let's spend a few minutes now, just thinking about what that will be like. What do you think about that—about what it will feel like to really know and understand yourself (or *"all parts of yourself"* if dissociation has been well *explained and accepted*) And tell me how that feels.

It may be hard for her to put it into words—but some youngsters just launch right in

Associating thoughts and feelings—often a new concept

They may find it difficult to put it into words, but you can offer subtle support as they find their way and begin to express their feelings.

Yes, it's a different feeling. And it's one that you will find easier, more and more comfortable as times goes on and you get even more comfortable within yourself. You'll be able to make better decisions, because lots of the unknowns are answered and you find yourself more and more aware of your life and your future.

"More and more ..." and "... comfortable ..." reinforced

And when you look back on it, in that future time, you can be very, very proud of yourself for the work that you have done, while helping yourself to get well. Because nobody can get well for you. Do you agree? (*Signals Yes*)

Establishing and reinforcing that sense of self-worth, and repeating that she has to do it for herself

So we'll be spending quite a lot of time together, over the next few months, as you realize your own worth. Because you are a really worthwhile person, and you can look forward to discovering that for yourself.

Positive future

I'll just be quiet again for a few moments, and then you can come out of hypnosis in your own way.

Offering her a little more time

That's right. Come back now, when you feel ready to do that.

Hello! That was a good session, wasn't it? (*Yes*) I thought so, too.

References

Bowlby, J. (1969) *Attachment and Loss*, Vol. I, Attachment, New York, NY: Basic Books

Crawford, H. (1995) "Brain dynamic shifts during hypnotic analgesia: Why can't we all eliminate pain?", *American Society of Clinical Hypnosis*, Chicago

Diegel, D. (1999) *The Developing Brain: Toward a neurobiology of interpersonal experience*, New York, NY: Guilford Press

Emerson, G. (2003) *Ego State Therapy*, Crown House Publishing, Wales

Francis, C. Y. and Houghton, L. A. (1996) "Use of hypnotherapy in gastrointestinal disorders", *European Journal of Gastroenterology and Hepatology*, Vol 8.

Gardner, G. G. and Olness, K. (1981, 1996) *Hypnosis and Hypnotherapy with Children*, 3rd edition, Guilford: Grunr & Stratton: New York

Herman, J (2001) *Trauma and Recovery: From Domestic Abuse to Political Terror*, Rivers Oram Press, London

Jevna, R. F. and Levitan, A. (1989) *No Time for Nonsense: Self-help for the seriously ill*, LuraMedia, San Diego, California

Johnson, C. and Webster, D. (2002) *Recrafting a life: Solutions for chronic pain and illness*, Brunner-Routledge, New York

Lakoff, G. and Johnson, M. (1980) *Metaphors We Live By*, University of Chicago Press, Chicago

Melzack, R. (1990) "Phantom limbs and concept of neuromatrix", *Trends in Neuroscience*, Vol. 13

Nijenhuis, E. (1999) *Somatoform Dissociation*, Assen, The Netherlands: van Gorcum and Co

Phillips, M. (2000) *Finding the Energy to Heal: How EMDR, hypnosis, TFT, imagery and body-focussed therapy can help restore mindbody health*, W. W. Norton, New York

Phillips, M and Frederick, C. (1995) *Hypnotherapy for Post-traumatic and Dissociative Conditions*; W.W. Norton, New York

Putnam, F.W. (1989) *Diagnosis and Treatment of Multiple Personality Disorder*, New York, NY: Guilford Press

Rossi, E (1986) *The Psychobiology of Mind-Body Healing*, New York, NY: W. W. Norton

Rossi, E (2002) *The Psychobiology of Gene expression: Neuroscience and Neurogenesis in Hypnosis and the Healing Arts*, Vol. 26.

Scaer, R. C. (2001) "The neurophysiology of dissociation and chronic disease", *Applied Psychophysiology and Biofeedback*, Vol. 26.

Sullivan, M. and Katon, W. (1993) "Somatization: The path between distress and somatic symptoms", *APS Bulletin*, Vol. 2.

van der Kolk (1994) "The body keeps the score: Memory and the evolving psychobiology of post-traumatic stress", Harvard Medical School Psychiatric Review.

Van der Kolk B. A. (2003) "The psychobiology of post-traumatic stress disorder", in Jaak Panksepp (ed.), *Textbook of Biological Psychiatry* (New York, NY: John Wiley & Sons).

Watkins J. G. and Watkins H. H. (1992) *Hypnosis and Ego State Therapy: Innovations in clinical hypnosis: A source book*, Vol. 10, Sarasota, FL: Professional Resource Exchange

Zarren, J. I. and Eimer, B. N. (2002) *Brief Cognitive Hypnosis; Facilitating the change of dysfunctional behavior*, Springer Publishing Company, New York

Zilberheld, B., Edelstein, M. G. and Araoz, D. (1986) *Hypnosis: question and answers*, W. W. Norton, New York

Index

Acute Traumatic Stress Disorder
    definition 77, viii
    denial 77
    new research in Israel 78
    numbing 84
    physiological response to trauma 86
    self-worth 84
        difference from self-esteem 84
Anxiety disorder 97
    conditioned 97
    free-floating 102
    reactive 97

Blending
    definition 140
    multiple blends 152
    power to choose 140
    reacting to outside world 143

Children
    child ego states—difference 159
    from abusive homes 159
    promise not to tell 163
        ways to get around it 164
Critical Incident Stress Disorder 90
    debriefing 91
    definition 90
    misperception 91

Debriefing 38, 91, 131
Denial 31, 34, 77, 78, 113, 114
Depression
    as part of PTSD 110
Disclosure 124, 125
Dissociative Disorders 119
    applying for a job 136
    child parts 122
    disclosure 124
    ego state approach 120
    ego-strengthening 131
        assertiveness 133
    hypnosis and dissociation 119
    maturing process 138
    safety and containment 119
    safety shields 128

Ego states viii, 9

Flashbacks
    and memories 51
    pain 21
Frederick, D. Claire 83, 108, 171

Goals 24, 52, 165
Grief and Bereavement 112
    acceptance 114
    anger 113
    bargaining 113
    children 116
    denial 113
    depression 114
    palliative care 117
    therapeutic abortion 115

Hyperarousal 41
Hypervigilance 36–38, 41, 81

Integration
    definition 148
    preparing 156
    various approaches 157
International Society for the Study of
    Trauma and Dissociation ix

Kübler-Ross, Dr Elisabeth 114

Mind-Body communication 5

Nijenhuis, Dr. Ellert 9
Numbering 77, 86

Pain
    and dissociation 1, 2, 13
    as emotion 5, 13
    chronic 24
    chronic pain syndrome 24, 26
    flashback pain 21
    intrusion and interference 5
    physical 17
    organic 19
    physiological 17
    psychological 5
    related to trauma 1
    similes, use of 4